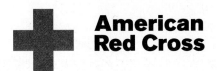

P9-DEL-503

A MediMedia USA Company

First Aid/CPR/AED for Schools and the Community

Important certification information

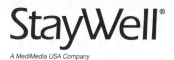

Composition by Graphic World
Printing/Binding by

StayWell
780 Township Line Rd.
Yardley, PA 19067

Library of Congress Cataloging-in-Publication Data

First aid/CPR/AED for schools and the community / American Red Cross.— 3rd ed.
    p. cm.
  Previous ed. has title: Community first aid & safety.
  Includes bibliographical references and index.
  ISBN 1-58480-300-2
 1. First aid in illness and injury. 2. CPR (First aid) 3. Automated external defibrillation. I. American Red Cross. II. Community first aid & safety.

RC86.7.C644 2006
616.02'52—dc22

2006001886

06 07 08 09 10 / 9 8 7 6 5 4 3 2 1

Preface

This is the third edition of the *American Red Cross First Aid/CPR/AED for Schools and the Community Participant's Manual.* This is a revised version of the previously published text under the title *Community First Aid and Safety.*

Content reflects the 2005 Consensus on Science for CPR and Emergency Cardiovascular Care (ECC) and the Guidelines 2005 for First Aid. This participant's manual features the latest automated external defibrillation (AED) information and skills. Chapters on asthma and epinephrine administration have been added. The design and content have been significantly updated with a new format for sidebars, boxes, skill sheets and more. A significant number of new photos have been introduced. Activities and quizzes are designed to make learning exciting and fun for students.

This participant's manual is part of an integral training program with certification available from your local American Red Cross chapter. CPR and AED certifications are valid for 1 year, while first aid certification is valid for 3 years. Contact your local American Red Cross at *www.redcross.org* for more information on how you can receive American Red Cross life-saving certification.

For more information on American Red Cross Health and Safety Services training and products, visit *www.redcross.org* or *www.shopstaywell.com.*

Acknowledgments

This manual is dedicated to the thousands of employees and volunteers of the American Red Cross who contribute their time and talent to supporting and teaching life-saving skills worldwide. And to the thousands of course participants and other readers who have decided to be prepared to take action when an emergency strikes.

We have endeavored to improve and polish this manual and course, which reflects the 2005 Consensus on Science for CPR and Emergency Cardiovascular Care (ECC) and Guidelines 2005 for First Aid. Many individuals shared in the development and revision process in various supportive, technical and creative ways. Each edition could not have been developed without the dedication and support of employees and volunteers.

The American Red Cross team for this third edition included—Ted T. Crites, CHES, Project Manager; Pat Bonifer, Director; Greg Stockton, Martha Chapin, Connie Harvey, Jeff Grebinoski, Don Lauritzen, Sandy Lovett and Marc Madden, Senior Associates; Adreania McMillian, Mark Schraf, John Thompson and Katherine Tunney, Associates; Greta Petrilla, Communications and Marketing Manager; and Betty Butler and Rhadames Avila, Administrative Assistants.

The StayWell team for this third edition included: Nancy Monahan, Senior Vice President; Bill Winneberger, Senior Director of Manufacturing; Paula Batt, Executive Director, Sales and Business Development; Reed Klanderud, Executive Director, Marketing and New Product Development; Shannon Bates, Managing Editor; Lorraine P. Coffey, Senior Developmental Editor; Amanda Land, Marketing Manager; and Stephanie Weidel, Senior Production Editor.

The American Red Cross and StayWell thank Allan Braslow, PhD, Robert Brennan, EdD, Anne Batcheller, RN, BSN and Irene F. Goodman, EdD of Goodman Research Group, Inc., Terry Georgia, Craig Reinertson, Casey M. Berg and Rick Brady for their contributions to this project.

The following members of the American Red Cross Advisory Council on First Aid and Safety (ACFAS) also provided guidance and review—

Georges C. Benjamin, MD, FACP
American Public Health Association
Washington, DC

Kim Dickerson, EMT-P, RN
Fort Myers, Florida

Jonathan L. Epstein, MEMS, NREMT-P
Northeast EMS, Inc.
Wakefield, Massachusetts

Paul Gannon, MS Ed, RN
West Seneca, New York

Susan Goekler, Ph.D., CHES
Tallmadge, Ohio

Claudia Hines, RN
St. Louis Park, Minnesota

James A. Judge, II, C.E.M.
Mt. Dora, Florida

Dawn O. Kleindorfer, MD
Department of Neurology
University of Cincinnati
Cincinnati, Ohio

David Markenson, MD, FAAP, EMT-P
Chief Pediatric Emergency Medicine
Maria Fareri Children's Hospital
Westchester Medical Center
Valhalla, New York

Edward V. Sargent, MPH, Ph.D., DABT
Merck & Co., Inc.
Two Merck Drive
P.O. Box 100, WS2F-45
Whitehouse Station, New Jersey

The American Red Cross would like to acknowledge members of the First Aid CPR/AED (r.06) Program Advisory Group for their guidance and review:

Anne E. Dinterman, Ed/HRD
Resources Assistant Director
Virginia Department of Transportation
American Red Cross
Colonial Virginia Chapter
Williamsburg, Virginia

Jody A. Eckler, M.S.
Director of Community Services
American Red Cross
Firelands Chapter
Sandusky, Ohio

Robert L. Harris, CFIAI
Associate Instructor, Clinical Education
Queen's Medical Center
American Red Cross
Hawaii State Chapter
Honolulu, Hawaii

Teresa A. May
Volunteer Instructor Trainer
American Red Cross
Greater Salt Lake Area Chapter
Salt Lake City, Utah

Cheryl J. Murray
Training Specialist
American Red Cross
Greater Milwaukee Chapter
Pewaukee, Wisconsin

Lynne M. Osborne, MA, EMT, I/C
Manager, Workplace Program
American Red Cross
Southeastern Michigan Chapter
Detroit, Michigan

Pedro M. Pares, MD
Professor of Health Sciences
University of Puerto Rico
Medical Sciences Campus
American Red Cross
Puerto Rico Chapter
San Juan, Puerto Rico

Angela K. Sehgal, EdD, ATC/L
Athletic Training/Sports Medicine
Education Program Coordinator
American Red Cross
Capital Area Chapter
Tallahassee, Florida

Thelma M. Specker, M.Ed. & M. Sc. Biology
Volunteer Instructor Trainer
American Red Cross
Southeastern Pennsylvania Chapter
Philadelphia, Pennsylvania

Jane M. Wiehe, RN
First Aid/CPR Training Coordinator
American Red Cross
Cincinnati Area Chapter
Cincinnati, Ohio

Table of Contents

About This Manual, ix

Health Precautions and Guidelines During First Aid Training, xi

Together We Prepare, xiii

Chapter 1: If Not YOU…Who?, 1

You and The Emergency Medical System, 2
Getting Permission to Give Care, 9
Skill Sheet: Removing Gloves, 12

Chapter 2: Taking Action: Emergency Action Steps, 15

Check, 16
Call, 17
Care, 19
Reaching and Moving an Ill or Injured Person: Do No Further Harm, 20

Chapter 3: Checking an Ill or Injured Person, 29

Checking a Conscious Person, 30
Checking an Unconscious Person, 32
Shock, 34
Skill Sheet: Checking a Conscious Person, 36
Skill Sheet: Checking an Unconscious Adult, 39
Skill Sheet: Checking an Unconscious Child, 40
Skill Sheet: Checking an Unconscious Infant, 42

Chapter 4: When Seconds Count, 45

Life-Threatening Emergencies, 45
Skill Sheet: Conscious Choking—Adult, 60
Skill Sheet: Conscious Choking—Child, 61
Skill Sheet: Conscious Choking—Infant, 62
Skill Sheet: How to Give a Rescue Breath—Adult, 63
Skill Sheet: Rescue Breathing—Child, 64
Skill Sheet: Rescue Breathing—Infant, 65

Chapter 5: Cardiac Emergencies, 67

Signals of a Heart Attack, 69
In Case of a Heart Attack, 71
Cardiac Emergencies In Children and Infants, 76
Using an AED—Adults, 80
Using an AED—Children, 81
Skill Sheet: CPR—Adult, 86
Skill Sheet: Unconscious Choking—Adult, 88
Skill Sheet: CPR—Child, 90
Skill Sheet: Unconscious Choking—Child, 92
Skill Sheet: CPR—Infant, 94
Skill Sheet: Unconscious Choking—Infant, 96
Skill Sheet: AED—Adult, 98
Skill Sheet: AED—Child, 100

Chapter 6: Injury Prevention, 103

Injuries, 103

Chapter 7: Soft Tissue Injuries: Cuts, Scrapes and Bruises, 111

Wounds, 112
Burns, 119
Special Situations, 121
Skill Sheet: Controlling External Bleeding, 126

Chapter 8: Injuries to Muscles, Bones and Joints, 129

Muscles, 130
Bones, 131
Joints, 131
Types of Injuries, 131
Skill Sheet: Applying an Anatomic Splint, 142
Skill Sheet: Applying a Soft Splint, 144
Skill Sheet: Applying a Rigid Splint, 146
Skill Sheet: Applying a Sling and Binder, 148

Chapter 9: Sudden Illness, 151

Recognizing Sudden Illness, 151
Caring for Sudden Illness, 152
Specific Sudden Illnesses, 152
Stroke, 157

Chapter 10: Poisoning, 161

Swallowed, Inhaled, Absorbed and Injected Poisons, 162
Checking the Scene for Poisoning, 163
General Care for Poisoning, 164
Special Care Considerations, 164

Chapter 11: Heat- or Cold-Related Emergencies, 175

Heat-Related Illness, 177
Cold-Related Illness, 178
Preventing Heat- and Cold-Related Emergencies, 180

Chapter 12: Special Situations and Circumstances, 183

Infants and Children, 183
Older Adults, 186
Emergency Childbirth, 188
People with Disabilities, 188
Language Barriers, 190
Crime Scenes and Hostile Situations, 191

Chapter 13: Asthma, 193

Asthma, 193
Skill Sheet: Assisting with Asthma Inhaler, 196

Chapter 14: Anaphylaxis and Epinephrine Auto-Injectors, 199

Anaphylaxis, 199
Skill Sheet: Assisting with an Epinephrine Auto-Injector, 202

Sources, 204

Index, 206

About This Manual

This manual has been designed to help you acquire the knowledge and skills you will need to effectively respond to emergency situations. The following pages point out some of the manual's special features including sidebars, boxes and skill sheets.

Sidebar—Feature articles called sidebars give you additional information about the material presented in the course and provide relevant background information. They appear in most chapters and have a pale yellow background. Sidebars feature historical and current information that relate to the chapter's content. You will not be tested on any information presented in these sidebars as part of the American Red Cross course completion requirements.

DID YOU KNOW?

HOW DISEASE SPREADS

Infectious diseases—those that can spread from one person to another—develop when germs invade the body and cause illness. The most common germs are bacteria and viruses.

Bacteria can live outside the body and do not depend on other organisms for life. The number of bacteria that infect humans is very small, but some can cause serious infections. These can be treated with medications called antibiotics.

Viruses depend on other organisms to live. Once in the body, they are hard to remove. Few medications can fight viruses. The body's immune system is the number one protection against infection.

Herpes simplex II virus.

Touching, Breathing and Biting
How do bacteria and viruses spread from one person to another? Through touching, breathing and biting.

You can become infected if you touch an infected person. This can happen when germs from the person's blood or other body fluids pass into your body through breaks or cuts in your skin or through the lining of your eyes, nose or mouth. You can also be infected when you touch an object that has been soiled by a person's blood or body fluids.

Some diseases, such as the common cold, are transmitted by droplets in the air we breathe. They are also passed on through contact with

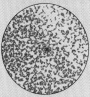

Streptococcus agalactia bacteria.

shared objects like spoons, doorknobs and pencils that have been exposed to the droplets. Fortunately, simply being exposed to these germs is usually not adequate for diseases to be transmitted.

Animals, including humans, can spread some diseases through bites. Contracting a disease from a bite is rare in any situation and uncomm[on] when giving first aid. Some[diseases] eases are spread more ea[sily] than others. Some of these[,] like the flu, can create dis[com]fort, but are often tempora[ry] and usually not serious for healthy adults.

Other germs can be more [seri]ous, such as hepatitis B vi[rus] (HBV), hepatitis C virus (HC[V)] and the human immunodef[i]ciency virus (HIV), which causes acquired immune d[efi]ciency syndrome (AIDS). Although very serious, the[y are] not easily transmitted and [are] not spread by casual cont[act] such as shaking hands. Th[e] primary way to transmit H[BV,] HCV or HIV during first aid care is through blood-to-b[lood] contact.

It Not YOU…Wh[o]

Box—Boxes contain crucial information that you need to know. They appear throughout the manual and have a red background. You may be tested on any information presented in a box as part of the American Red Cross course completion requirements.

Consider the following:
- Over 40 million injury-related visits were made to U.S. hospital emergency departments in 2003.
- Injuries resulted in more than 160,000 deaths in the U.S. in 2003.
- Unintentional injuries cause most childhood deaths.
- More than 70 million people in the United States have cardiovascular disease.
- Cardiovascular disease causes about 700,000 deaths in the United States each year.[4] That accounts

for over 33 percent of all U.S. deaths annually!
- About 700,000 Americans have strokes each year and of these, more than 160,000 die from the stroke.

Each time a person is injured or experiences a sudden illness, such as a heart attack or a stroke, someone has to do something to help. Someday it may be you. Everyone should know what to do in an emergency. You should know who to call, what care to provide and how to give first aid until

emergency medical help arrives. Everyone should know first aid, but even if you have not had any first aid training you can still help in an emergency.

YOU AND THE EMERGENCY MEDICAL SYSTEM

You play a major role in making the emergency medical services (EMS) system work effectively. The EMS system is a network of police, fire and medical personnel, as well as other community resources.

Your role in the EMS system includes four basic steps:

Step 1. Recognize that an Emergency Exists

Emergencies can happen to anyone, anywhere. Before you can give help, however, you must be able to recognize an emergency. You may realize that an emergency has occurred only if something unusual attracts your attention. For example, you may become aware of unusual noises, sights, odors and appearances or behaviors.

Noises that may signal an emergency include screaming or calls for help; breaking glass, crashing metal or screeching tires; a change in the sound made by machinery or equipment; or sudden, loud noises, such as the sound of collapsing buildings or falling ladders.

Signals of an emergency that you may see include a car that has run off the road, downed electrical wires, a person lying motionless, spilled medication, fallen boxes, smoke or fire (Fig. 1-2, A-C).

Many odors are part of our everyday lives. Examples include gasoline fumes at the gas station, chlorine at a swimming pool, bleach at home and chemicals at a refinery. However, when these are stronger than usual, there

CRITICAL FACTS

RECOGNIZING EMERGENCIES

Your senses—hearing, sight and smell—may help you recognize an emergency. Emergencies are often signaled by something unusual that catches your attention. Examples include:

Unusual Noises
- Screaming, yelling, moaning or calling for help.
- Breaking glass, crashing metal or screeching tires.
- Sudden, loud or unidentifiable sounds.
- Unusual silence.

Unusual Sights
- Stopped vehicle on the roadside.
- Broken glass.
- Overturned pot in the kitchen.
- Spilled medicine container.
- Downed electrical wires.
- Sparks, smoke or fire.

Unusual Odors
- Odors that are stronger than usual.
- Unrecognizable odors.
- Inappropriate odors.

Unusual Appearances or Behaviors
- Unconsciousness.
- Confused or unusual behavior.
- Trouble breathing.
- Clutching chest or throat.
- Slurred, confused or hesitant speech.
- Unexplainable confusion or drowsiness.
- Sweating for no apparent reason.
- Uncharacteristic skin color.
- Inability to move a body part.

Skill Sheets—At the end of certain chapters, Skill Sheets give step-by-step directions for performing specific skills. Learning specific skills that you will need to give appropriate care for victims of sudden illness or injury is an important part of this course. Photographs enhance each Skill Sheet. Skill Sheets are presented on a taupe background, with their titles in white.

Applying an Anatomic Splint

CHECK the scene for safety. **CHECK** the injured person following standard precautions. **CALL** 9-1-1 or the local emergency number if necessary. To **CARE** for a person who has an injured limb—

STEP 1
Obtain consent.

STEP 2
Support the injured body part above and below the site of the injury.

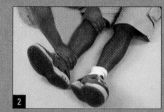
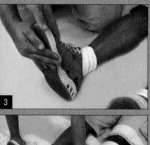

STEP 3
Check for feeling, warmth and color.

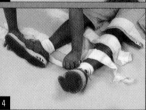

STEP 4
Place several folded triangular bandages above and below the injured body part.

142 | First Aid/CPR/AED for Schools and the Community

Health Precautions and Guidelines During First Aid Training

The American Red Cross has trained millions of people in first aid and cardiopulmonary resuscitation (CPR) using manikins as training aids.

The Red Cross follows widely accepted guidelines for cleaning and decontaminating training manikins. **If these guidelines are adhered to, the risk of any kind of disease transmission during training is extremely low.**

To help minimize the risk of disease transmission, you should follow some basic health precautions and guidelines while participating in training. You should take precautions if you have a condition that would increase your risk or other participants' risk of exposure to infections. Request a separate training manikin if you—

- Have an acute condition, such as a cold, a sore throat, or cuts or sores on the hands or around your mouth.
- Know you are seropositive (have had a positive blood test) for hepatitis B surface antigen (HBsAg), indicating that you are currently infected with the hepatitis B virus.*
- Know you have a chronic infection indicated by long-term seropositivity (long-term positive blood tests) for the hepatitis B surface antigen (HBsAg)* or a positive blood test for anti-HIV (that is, a positive test for antibodies to HIV, the virus that causes many severe infections including AIDS).
- Have had a positive blood test for hepatitis C (HCV).
- Have a type of condition that makes you unusually likely to get an infection.

To obtain information about testing for individual health status, visit the CDC Web site at: *www.cdc.gov/ncidod/diseases/hepatitis/c/faq.htm*

After a person has had an acute hepatitis B infection, he or she will no longer test positive for the surface antigen but will test positive for the hepatitis B antibody (anti-HBs). Persons who have been vaccinated for hepatitis B will also test positive for the hepatitis antibody. A positive test for the hepatitis B antibody (antiHBs) should not be confused with a positive test for the hepatitis B surface antigen (HBsAG).

---

*A person with hepatitis B infection will test positive for the hepatitis B surface antigen (HBsAg). Most persons infected with hepatitis B will get better within a period of time. However, some hepatitis B infections will become chronic and will linger for much longer. These persons will continue to test positive for HBsAg. Their decision to participate in CPR training should be guided by their physician.

If you decide you should have your own manikin, ask your instructor if he or she can provide one for you to use. You will **not** be asked to explain why in your request. The manikin will not be used by anyone else until it has been cleaned according to the recommended end-of-class decontamination procedures. Because the number of manikins available for class use is limited, the more advance notice you give, the more likely it is that you can be provided a separate manikin.

Some people are sensitive to certain allergens and may have an allergic reaction. If you start experiencing skin redness, rash, hives, itching, runny nose, sneezing, itchy eyes, scratchy throat or signs of asthma, wash your hands immediately. If conditions persist or you experience a severe reaction, stop training and seek medical attention right away.

Guidelines

In addition to taking the precautions regarding manikins, you can further protect yourself and other participants from infection by following these guidelines:

- Wash your hands thoroughly before participating in class activities.
- Do not eat, drink, use tobacco products or chew gum during class when manikins are used.
- Clean the manikin properly before use.
- For some manikins, this means vigorously wiping the manikin's face and the inside of its mouth with a clean gauze pad soaked with either a fresh solution of liquid chlorine bleach and water (¼ cup sodium hypochlorite per gallon of tap water) or rubbing alcohol. The surfaces should remain wet for at least 1 minute before they are wiped dry with a second piece of clean, absorbent material.
- For other manikins, it means changing the manikin's face. Your instructor will provide you with instructions for cleaning the type of manikin used in your class.
- Follow the guidelines provided by your instructor when practicing skills such as clearing a blocked airway with your finger.

Physical Stress and Injury

Successful course completion requires full participation in classroom and skill sessions, as well as successful performance in skill and knowledge evaluations. Due to the nature of the skills in this course, you will be participating in strenuous activities, such as performing CPR on the floor. If you have a medical condition or disability that will prevent you from taking part in the skills practice sessions, please let your instructor know so that accommodations can be made. If you are unable to participate fully in the course, you may "audit" the course and participate as much as you can or desire. In order to audit a course, you must let the instructor know before the training begins. Be aware that you will *not* be eligible to receive a course completion certificate unless you participate fully and meet all course objectives and prerequisites.

Together We Prepare

The American Red Cross mission is to provide relief to victims of disaster and help people prevent, prepare for and respond to emergencies. But we need your help. There are five actions that every organization, individual and family should take to better prepare themselves for an emergency or disaster, these include—

- **Make a plan.** Everyone should design a Family Disaster Plan. The Family Disaster Plan focuses on both families and individuals.
- **Build a kit.** For your home and workplace, assemble a Disaster Supplies Kit, which contains items that you may need if you are 1) confined to your home or place of work for an extended period (e.g., after a disaster or winter storm) or 2) told to evacuate on short notice.
- **Get trained.** Participate in first aid, CPR and AED training and attend Red Cross Community Disaster Education presentations.
- **Volunteer.** Give your time through volunteering.
- **Give blood.** Become a regular and frequent blood donor to ensure a blood supply that meets all needs, all of the time.

For more information visit *www.redcross.org*

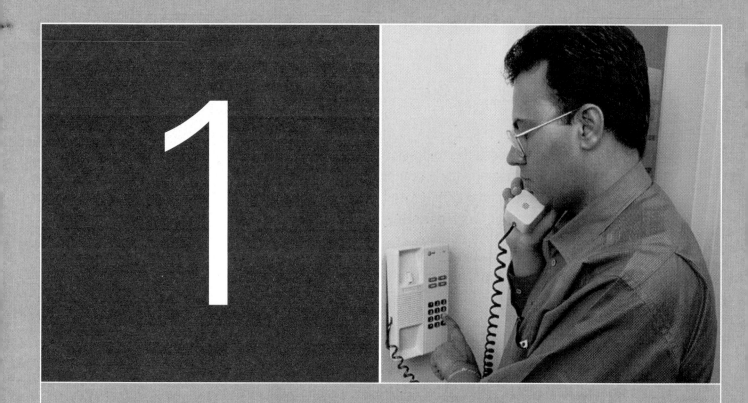

1

Everyone should know first aid.

Chapter 1

If Not YOU...Who?

You're late for the party. Why did you say you'd get there by 7 o'clock? Better stop at the convenience store for the drinks instead of the grocery store. That will save a few minutes. Why are all those people standing around over there? Oh no! It's the person who works here... You leave the car and see the young man lying on his back, looking dazed and holding his head. Even though a crowd has gathered, no one is helping him. They're just looking at each other. He needs help from someone. That someone could be you.

If placed in the above situation, would you step forward to help? "I hope I never have to," is what you are probably thinking. However, given the number of injuries and sudden illnesses that occur in the United States each year (Fig. 1-1), you might have to deal with an emergency situation someday.

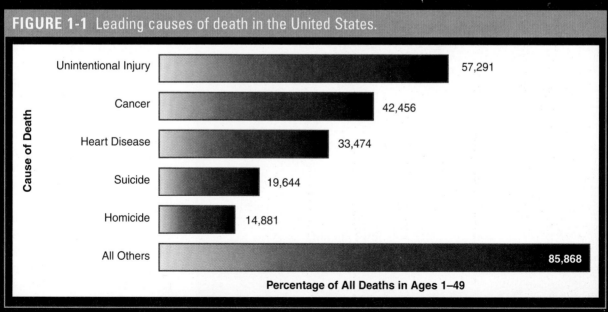

FIGURE 1-1 Leading causes of death in the United States.

Data Source: National Center for Health Statistics, National Vital Statistics System

Consider the following:

- Over 40 million injury-related visits were made to U.S. hospital emergency departments in 2003.
- Injuries resulted in more than 160,000 deaths in the U.S. in 2003.
- Unintentional injuries cause most childhood deaths.
- More than 70 million people in the U.S. have cardiovascular disease.
- Cardiovascular disease causes about 700,000 deaths in the U.S. each year. That accounts for over 33 percent of all U.S. deaths annually!
- About 700,000 Americans have strokes each year and of these, more than 160,000 die from the stroke.

Each time a person is injured or experiences a sudden illness, such as a heart attack or a stroke, someone has to do something to help. Someday it may be you. Everyone should know what to do in an emergency. You should know who to call, what care to give and how to give first aid until emergency medical help arrives. Everyone should know first aid, but even if you have not had any first aid training you can still help in an emergency.

YOU AND THE EMERGENCY MEDICAL SYSTEM

You play a major role in making the emergency medical services (EMS) system work effectively. The EMS system is a network of police, fire and medical personnel, as well as other community resources.

Your role in the EMS system includes four basic steps:

Step 1. Recognize that an Emergency Exists

Emergencies can happen to anyone, anywhere. Before you can give help, however, you must be able to recognize an emergency. You may realize that an emergency has occurred only if something unusual attracts your attention. For example, you may become aware of unusual noises, sights, odors and appearances or behaviors.

Noises that may signal an emergency include screaming or calls for help; breaking glass, crashing metal or screeching tires; a change in the sound made by machinery or equipment; or sudden, loud noises, such as the sound of collapsing buildings or falling ladders.

Signals of an emergency that you may see include a car that has run off the road, downed electrical wires, a person lying motionless, spilled medication, fallen boxes, smoke or fire (Fig. 1-2, A-C).

Many odors are part of our everyday lives. Examples include gasoline fumes at the gas station, chlorine at a swimming pool, bleach at home and chemicals at a refinery. However, when these are stronger than usual, there

---

CRITICAL FACTS

RECOGNIZING EMERGENCIES

Your senses—hearing, sight and smell—may help you recognize an emergency. Emergencies are often signaled by something unusual that catches your attention. Examples include—

Unusual Sights
- Stopped vehicle on the roadside
- Broken glass
- Overturned pot in the kitchen
- Spilled medicine container
- Downed electrical wires
- Sparks, smoke or fire

Unusual Appearances or Behaviors
- Unconsciousness
- Confused or unusual behavior
- Trouble breathing
- Clutching chest or throat
- Slurred, confused or hesitant speech
- Unexplainable confusion or drowsiness

- Sweating for no apparent reason
- Uncharacteristic skin color
- Inability to move a body part

Unusual Odors
- Odors that are stronger than usual
- Unrecognizable odors
- Inappropriate odors

Unusual Noises
- Screaming, yelling, moaning or calling for help
- Breaking glass, crashing metal or screeching tires
- Sudden, loud or unidentifiable sounds
- Unusual silence

FIGURE 1-2, A-C Unusual sights may indicate an emergency.

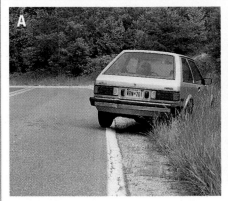
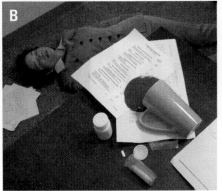
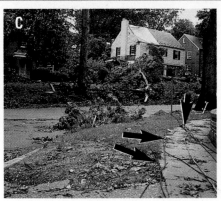

may be an emergency. Also, an unusual odor may mean something is wrong. Put your own safety first. Leave the area if there is an unusual or very strong odor, since some fumes are poisonous.

It may be difficult to tell if someone is behaving strangely or if something is wrong, especially if you do not know the person. Sometimes, though, there is little doubt. For example, if you see someone suddenly collapse, slip or fall, there is a good chance the person might need help (Fig. 1-3).

Other signals of a possible emergency might not be as easy to recognize. These include trouble breathing, confused behavior, unusual skin color and signals of pain and discomfort such as clutching the chest or throat, being doubled over or facial expressions indicating something is wrong.

Step 2. Decide to Act

Once you recognize an emergency has occurred, you must decide whether to help and what to do. There are many ways you can help in an emergency. In order to help, you must act.

Whether or not you have had first aid training, being faced with an emergency will probably bring out mixed feelings. While wanting to help, you may also feel hesitant or want to back away from the situation. These feelings are personal and real. The

In order to help, you must act.

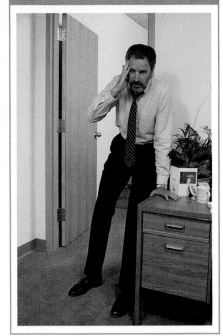

FIGURE 1-3 Unusual behavior is often a signal that something is wrong.

decision to act is yours and yours alone.

Sometimes, even though people recognize that an emergency has occurred, they fail to act. The most common factors that keep people from responding are—

- **The presence of other people.** If several people are standing around, it might not be easy to tell if anyone is giving first aid. Always ask if you can help. Just because there is a crowd does not mean someone is caring for the ill or injured person. In fact, you may be the only one on the scene who knows first aid.

Although you may feel embarrassed about coming forward in front of other people, this should not stop you from offering help. Someone has to take action in an emergency and it may have to be you.

If others are already giving care, ask if you can help. If bystanders do not appear to be helping, tell them how to help. You can ask them to call 9-1-1 or the local emergency number, meet the ambulance and direct it to your location, keep the area free of onlookers and traffic or help give care (Fig. 1-4). You might send them for blankets or other supplies.

THE EMS SYSTEM

The Emergency Medical Services (EMS) system is a network of community resources in which you play an important part.

The system begins when a responsible citizen like you recognizes that an emergency exists and decides to take action. You call 9-1-1 or the local emergency number for help. The EMS dispatcher answers the call and uses the information you give to determine what help is needed. A team of emergency personnel gives care at the scene and transports the ill or injured person to the hospital where emergency department staff and a variety of other professionals take over.

Early arrival of emergency personnel increases a person's chances of surviving a life-threatening emergency. Whether you know first aid or not, calling 9-1-1 or the local emergency number is the most important action you can take.

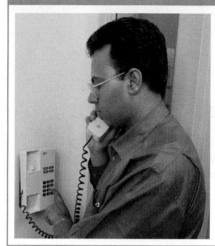

FIGURE 1-4 Bystanders can help you respond to an emergency by calling 9-1-1.

- **Being unsure of the ill or injured person's condition.** Because most emergencies happen in or near the home, you are more likely to find yourself giving care to a family member or a friend than to someone you do not know. However, you may be faced with an

You are more likely to care for a loved one than for someone you don't know.

emergency situation involving a stranger and you might feel uneasy about helping someone you do not know. For example, the person may be much older or much younger than you, be of a different gender or race, have a disabling condition, be of a different status at work or be the victim of a crime.

Sometimes, people who have been injured or become suddenly ill may act strangely or be uncooperative. The injury or illness, stress or other factors, such as the effects of drugs, alcohol or medications, may make people unpleasant or angry. Do not take this behavior personally. If you feel at all threatened by the person's behavior, leave the immediate area and call 9-1-1 or the local emergency number for help.

- **The type of injury or illness.** An injury or illness may sometimes be very unpleasant. Blood, vomit, bad odors, deformed body parts or torn or burned skin can be very upsetting. You may have to turn away for a moment and take a few deep breaths to get control of your feelings before you can give care. If you are still unable to give first aid, you can help in other ways, such as volunteering to call 9-1-1 or the local emergency number.

- **Fear of catching a disease.** Today, many people worry about the possibility of being infected with a disease while giving first aid. Although it is possible for diseases to be transmitted in a first aid situation, it is extremely unlikely that you will catch a disease this way. For more information on disease transmission, see "How Disease Spreads" and "Preventing Disease Transmission" later in this chapter.

HOW DISEASE SPREADS

Infectious diseases—those that can spread from one person to another—develop when germs invade the body and cause illness. The most common germs are bacteria and viruses.

Bacteria can live outside the body and do not depend on other organisms for life. The number of bacteria that infect humans is very small, but some can cause serious infections. These can be treated with medications called *antibiotics*.

Viruses depend on other organisms to live. Once in the body, they are hard to remove. Few medications can fight viruses. The body's immune system is its number one protection against infection.

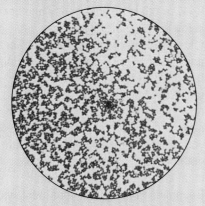

Streptococcus agalactia bacteria.

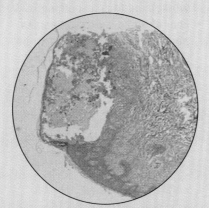

Herpes simplex II virus.

Touching, Breathing and Biting
How do bacteria and viruses spread from one person to another? Through touching, breathing and biting.

You can become infected if you touch an infected person. This can happen when germs from the person's blood or other body fluids pass into your body through breaks or cuts in your skin or through the lining of your eyes, nose or mouth. You can also be infected when you touch an object that has been soiled by a person's blood or body fluids.

Some diseases, such as the common cold, are transmitted by droplets in the air we breathe. They are also passed on through contact with shared objects like spoons, doorknobs and pencils that have been exposed to the droplets. Fortunately, simply being exposed to these germs is usually not adequate for diseases to be transmitted.

Animals, including humans, can spread some diseases through bites. Contracting a disease from a bite is rare in any situation and uncommon when giving first aid. Some diseases are spread more easily than others. Some of these, like the flu, can create discomfort, but are often temporary and usually not serious for healthy adults.

Other germs can be more serious, such as hepatitis B virus (HBV), hepatitis C virus (HCV) and the human immunodeficiency virus (HIV), which causes acquired immune deficiency syndrome (AIDS). Although very serious, they are not easily transmitted and are not spread by casual contact, such as shaking hands. The primary way to transmit HBV, HCV or HIV during first aid care is through blood-to-blood contact.

- **Fear of doing something wrong.** People react differently in emergencies. Whether trained in first aid or not, some people are afraid of doing the wrong thing and making matters worse. If you are not sure what to do, call 9-1-1 or the local emergency number. The worst thing to do is nothing.
- **Fear of being sued.** Sometimes people worry that they might be sued for giving first aid. In fact, lawsuits against people who give emergency care at a scene of an accident are highly unusual and rarely successful. All 50 states have enacted "Good Samaritan" laws that protect people who willingly give first aid without accepting anything in return. So you can help without worrying about lawsuits. For more on Good Samaritan laws, see "What Everyone Should Know About Good Samaritan Laws" later in this chapter.
- **Being unsure of when to call 9-1-1.** People sometimes are afraid to call 9-1-1 because they are not sure that the situation is a real emergency and do not want to waste the time of the emergency medical services.

Your decision to act in an emergency should be guided by your own values and by your knowledge of the risks that may be present. However, even if you decide not to give first aid, you should at least call 9-1-1 or the local emergency number to get emergency medical help.

Step 3. Activate the EMS System

Activating the EMS system by calling 9-1-1 or the local emergency number is the most important step you can take in an emergency. Know your local emergency number. Remember, some facilities, such as hotels, office and university buildings and some stores, require you to dial a 9 or some other number to get an outside line before you dial 9-1-1. Also, some areas without access to a 9-1-1 system use a local emergency number instead. Becoming familiar with your local system is important because the rapid arrival of emergency medical help greatly increases a person's chances of surviving a life-threatening emergency (Fig. 1-5, A-C).

PREVENTING DISEASE TRANSMISSION

By following some basic guidelines you can greatly decrease your risk of getting or transmitting an infectious disease while giving first aid—

- Avoid contact with blood and other body fluids when possible.
- Use protective breathing barriers, when possible, for any emergency situation requiring you to give rescue breaths.
- Use a bandage to cover any cuts, sores, scrapes or skin conditions you may have.
- Use barriers, such as disposable gloves, between the person's blood or body fluids and yourself.
- Do not eat, drink or touch your mouth, nose or eyes when giving first aid or before you wash your hands.
- Avoid handling any of your personal items, such as pens or combs, while giving care or before you wash your hands.
- Do not touch objects that may be soiled with blood.
- Be prepared by having a first aid kit handy and stocked with protective equipment and supplies.
- Wash your hands thoroughly with soap and warm running water when you have finished giving care, even if you wore disposable gloves.
  - Turn on warm water.
  - Wet hands with water.
  - Apply liquid soap to hands.
  - Rub your hands together vigorously for at least 15 seconds, covering all surfaces of the hands and fingers.
    - Use soap and warm running water.
    - Scrub nails by rubbing them against the palms of your hands.
  - Rinse your hands with water.
  - Dry your hands thoroughly with a paper towel.
  - Turn off the faucet using the paper towel.
- Tell EMS personnel at the scene or your doctor if you have come into direct contact with an ill or injured person's body fluids.

FIGURE 1-5, A-C Calling 9-1-1 or your local emergency number is important because getting emergency help fast greatly increases a person's chances of survival.

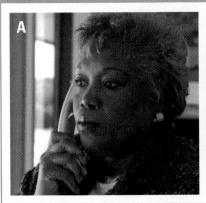
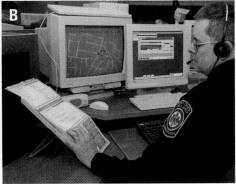
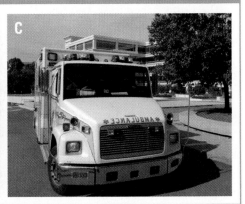

WHAT EVERYONE SHOULD KNOW ABOUT GOOD SAMARITAN LAWS

Are there laws to protect you when you provide help in an emergency situation?

Yes, all 50 states have enacted Good Samaritan laws, which give legal protection to people who willingly provide emergency care to ill or injured persons without accepting anything in return.

Good Samaritan laws usually protect citizens who act the same way that a "reasonable and prudent person" would if that person were in the same situation. For example, a reasonable and prudent person would—

- Move a person only if the person's life were in danger.
- Ask a conscious person for permission before giving care.
- Check the person for life-threatening conditions before giving further care.
- Call 9-1-1 or the local emergency number.
- Continue to give care until more highly trained personnel arrive.

Good Samaritan laws were developed to encourage people to help others in emergency situations. They require the "Good Samaritan" to use common sense and a reasonable level of skill, and to provide only the type of emergency first aid for which he or she is trained. They assume each person would do his or her best to save a life or prevent further injury.

Good Samaritan Protection in Lawsuits

Non-professionals who respond to emergencies, also called "lay responders," are rarely sued for helping in an emergency. However, Good Samaritan laws protect the responder from financial responsibility. In cases in which a lay responder's actions were deliberately negligent or reckless or when the responder abandoned the person after starting care, the courts have ruled Good Samaritan laws do not protect the responder.

If you are interested in finding out about your state's Good Samaritan laws, contact a legal professional or check with your local library.

HIV, AIDS AND YOU

The Disease

Acquired immune deficiency syndrome (AIDS) is a condition caused by HIV. When HIV gets into the body, it damages the immune systems that are supposed to fight infection. Eventually, the weakened immune systems allow certain types of infections to develop. The virus can grow quietly for months or even years. People infected with HIV might not feel or look sick. People with AIDS eventually develop life-threatening infections, which can cause them to die. Because there is currently no vaccine against HIV, prevention is still the best tool.

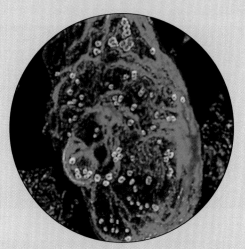

Human immunodeficiency virus (HIV).

Transmission During First Aid

The two most likely ways for HIV to be transmitted during first aid care would be through—

- **Unprotected direct contact with infected blood.** This type of transmission could happen if infected blood or body fluids from one person entered another person's body at a correct entry site. For example, a responder could contract HIV if the infected person's blood splashed in the responder's eye or if the responder directly touched the infected person's body fluids.
- **Unprotected indirect contact with infected blood.** This type of transmission could happen if a person touched an object that contained the blood or other body fluids of an infected person, and that infected blood or other body fluid entered the body through a correct entry site. For example, HIV could be transmitted if a responder picked up a blood-soaked bandage with a bare hand and the infected blood entered the responder's hand through a cut in the skin.

The virus cannot enter through the skin unless there is a cut or break in the skin. Even then, the possibility of infection is very low unless there is direct contact for a lengthy period of time. Saliva is not known to transmit HIV.

First Aid Precautions

The likelihood of HIV transmission during a first aid situation is very low. Always give care in ways that protect you and the person from disease transmission. For precaution details, see "Preventing Disease Transmission" on page 6.

Testing

If you think you have put yourself at risk, get tested. A readily available test will tell whether your body is producing antibodies in response to the virus. If you are not sure whether you should be tested, call your doctor, the public health department, an AIDS service organization or the AIDS hotline listed below and talk to them.

Hotline

If you have any questions, call the Centers for Disease Control and Prevention (CDC) national AIDS hotline at 1-800-342-2437, 24 hours a day, 7 days a week or the SIDA hotline (Spanish) at 1-800-344-7432, 24 hours a day, 7 days a week. TTY/TDD service is available at 1-800-243-7889, Monday through Friday, 10 a.m.-10 p.m., EST. Or call your local or state health department.

CLEANING UP A BLOOD SPILL

If a blood spill occurs—
- Clean up the spill immediately or as soon as possible after the spill occurs (Fig. 1-6).
- Use disposable gloves and other personal protective equipment when cleaning spills.
- Wipe up the spill with paper towels or other absorbent material.
- After the area has been wiped up, flood the area with a solution of approximately 1½ cups of liquid chlorine bleach to 1 gallon of fresh water (1 part bleach per 10 parts water), and allow it to stand for at least 10 minutes.
- Dispose of the contaminated material used to clean up the spill in a labeled biohazard container.

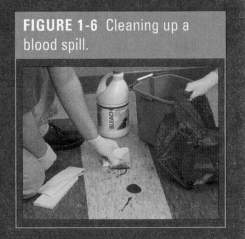

FIGURE 1-6 Cleaning up a blood spill.

Step 4. Give Care Until Help Arrives

This manual and the American Red Cross First Aid/CPR/AED for Schools and the Community course will provide you with the information and skills you need to give care to a person in an emergency medical situation.

The Difference Between Life and Death. If you are prepared for unforeseen emergencies, you can help ensure that care begins as soon as possible for yourself, your family and your fellow citizens. If you are trained in first aid, you can give help that can save a life in the first few minutes of an emergency. First aid can be the difference between life and death.

Often, it makes the difference between complete recovery and permanent disability. By knowing what to do and acting on that knowledge, you can make a difference.

GETTING PERMISSION TO GIVE CARE

You may want to care for an injured or ill person, but before giving first aid you must have the person's permission. This permission is referred to as "consent." To get permission you must tell the person who you are, how much training you have, what you think is wrong and what you plan to do. Only then can a conscious person give you permission to give care.

Do not give care to a conscious person who refuses it. If the conscious person is an infant or child, permission to give care should be obtained from a parent or guardian when one is available. If the condition is life threatening, permission is implied if a parent or guardian is not present. If the parent or guardian is present but does not give consent, do not give care. Instead, call 9-1-1 or the local emergency number.

Permission is also implied if you come upon a person who is unconscious or unable to respond. This means you can assume that if the person could respond, he or she would agree to care.

BE PREPARED

- Keep medical information about you and your family in a handy place, such as on the refrigerator door or in your car's glove compartment. Keep medical and insurance records up to date.

- Most communities are served by an emergency 9-1-1 telephone number. If your community does not operate on a 9-1-1 system, look up the numbers for the police, fire department and EMS. Emergency numbers are usually listed in the front of the telephone book. Know the number for the Poison Control Center, 800-222-1222, and post it on or near your telephones. Teach everyone in your home how and when to use these numbers.

- Keep all emergency telephone numbers in a handy place, such as by the telephone or in the first aid kit. Include home and work numbers of family members and friends. Be sure to keep both lists current.

- Keep a first aid kit handy in your home, car, workplace and recreation area.

- Learn and practice cardiopulmonary resuscitation (CPR) and first aid skills.

- Learn how to use an automated external defibrillator (AED) for victims of sudden cardiac arrest.

- Make sure your house or apartment number is easy to read. Numerals are easier to read than spelled-out numbers.

- Wear a medical ID bracelet or necklace if you have a potentially serious medical condition, such as epilepsy, diabetes, heart disease or allergies.

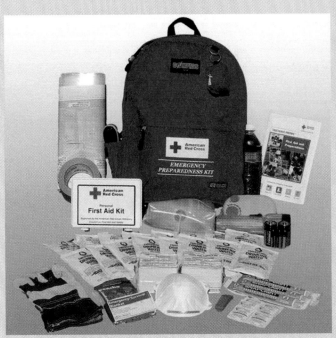

Deluxe Emergency Preparedness Kit

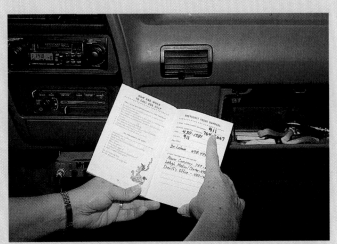

Keep important information in handy places such as your car's glove compartment.

Removing Gloves

STEP 1

Partially remove the first glove.

- Pinch the glove at the wrist, being careful to touch only the glove's outside surface.
- Pull the glove toward the fingertips without completely removing it.
- The glove is now partly inside out.

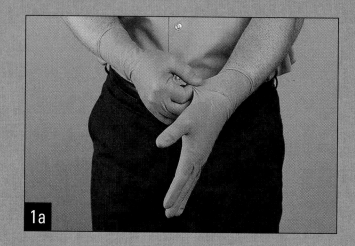

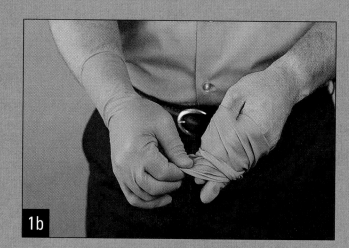

STEP 2

Remove the second glove.

- With your partially gloved hand, pinch the outside surface of the second glove.
- Pull the second glove toward the fingertips until it is inside out, and then remove it completely.

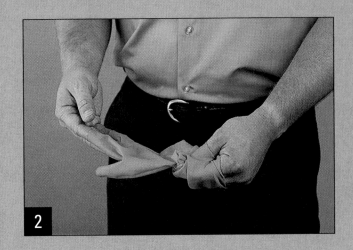

STEP 3

Finish removing both gloves.

- Grasp both gloves with your free hand.
- Touch only the clean interior surface of the glove.

STEP 4

After removing both gloves—

- Discard gloves in an appropriate container.
- Wash your hands thoroughly.

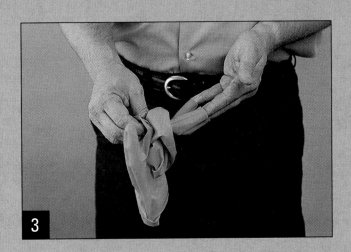

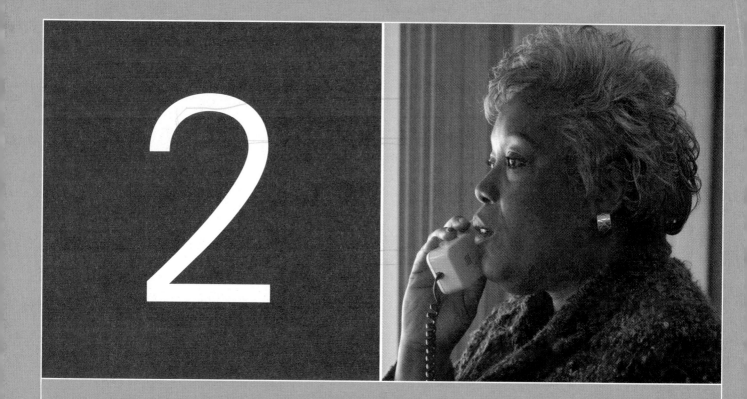

2

CHECK
CALL
CARE

Chapter 2

Taking Action:
Emergency Action Steps

It's 9:30 on a Saturday morning. The sudden sounds outside are close together but very clear—a screech of brakes, a thud and a shrill scream. You are out the door and onto the sidewalk before you have time to think about it. Maria and Rose have been playing out there!

People are running from all over. Your eyes take it in—the twisted bike, the van in the middle of the street and the child lying on the pavement. His left leg looks funny and there's blood on the pavement, but at least he's alive. He's moaning and crying. A man is staring at the boy. "He just came out of nowhere," he stammers. "All of the sudden, there he was, right in front of the van." The boy is obviously hurt. What should you do?

So far, you have learned that you can make a difference in an emergency. You may even save a life. You now know how to recognize an emergency. You have learned that the worst thing you can do is nothing and that deciding to get involved can be hard for anyone—not just you. You also know some things you can do to help.

Even so, when an emergency happens, you may feel confused. Fortunately, by learning first aid, you can train yourself to stay calm and think before you act.

If you find yourself in an emergency situation, you should always follow three basic emergency action steps—

1. **CHECK** the scene and the person.
2. **CALL** 9-1-1 or the local emergency number.
3. **CARE** for the person.

CHECK

Before you can help an ill or injured person, you must make sure the scene is safe for you and any bystanders (Fig. 2-1). Look the scene over and try to answer these questions—

- **Is it safe?** Check for anything unsafe, such as spilled chemicals, traffic, fire, escaping steam, downed electrical lines, smoke or extreme weather. Avoid going into confined areas with no ventilation or fresh air; places where there might be poisonous gas; collapsed structures; or places where natural gas, propane or other substances could explode. Such areas should only be entered by responders who have special training and equipment, such as respirators and self-contained breathing apparatus.

  If these or other dangers threaten, do not go near the ill or injured person. Stay at a safe distance and call 9-1-1 or the local emergency number immediately. If the scene is still unsafe after you call, do not enter. Keep yourself safe from danger. Dead or injured heroes are no help to anyone! Leave dangerous situations to professionals like firefighters and police. Once they make the scene safe, you can offer to help.

- **What happened?** Look for clues to what caused the emergency and how the person might be injured. Nearby objects, such as a fallen ladder, broken glass or a spilled bottle of medicine, may give you information. Your check of the scene may be the only way to tell what happened.

- **How many people are involved?** Look carefully for more than one person. You might not spot everyone at first. If one person is bleeding or screaming, you might not notice an unconscious person. It is also easy to overlook an infant or a small child. In an emergency with more than one victim, you may need to prioritize care (in other words, decide who needs help first).

- **Is there immediate danger involved?** Do not move a seriously injured person unless there is an immediate danger, such as fire, flood or poisonous gas; you have to reach another person who may have a more serious injury or illness; or you need to move the injured person to give proper care. If you must move the person, do it as quickly and carefully as possible. If there is no danger, tell the person not to move. Tell any bystanders not to move the person.

- **Is anyone else available to help?** You have already learned that the presence of bystanders does not mean that a person is receiving

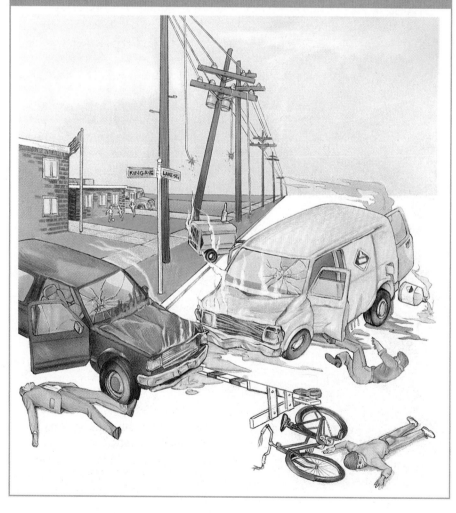

FIGURE 2-1 Check the scene for anything that may threaten the safety of you, the injured people and bystanders. Can you identify the hazards shown?

help. You may have to ask them to help. Bystanders may be able to tell you what happened or direct you to the nearest telephone. If a family member, friend or co-worker is present, he or she may know if the person is ill or has a medical condition.

The ill or injured person may be too upset to answer your questions. A child may be especially frightened. Anyone who awakens after having been unconscious for a few minutes may also be frightened. Bystanders can also help comfort the person and others at the scene. Parents or guardians who are present may be able to calm a frightened child. They can also tell you if a child has a medical condition.

- **What is wrong?** When you reach the person, you must try to find out what is wrong. Look for signals that may indicate a life-threatening emergency. First, check to see if the ill or injured person is conscious (Fig. 2-2). Sometimes this is obvious. The person may be able to speak to you. He or she may be moaning, crying, making some other noise or moving around. If the person is conscious, reassure him or her and try to find out what happened.

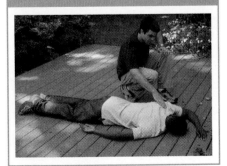

FIGURE 2-2 When you reach the person, first check to see if he or she is conscious.

If the person is lying on the ground, silent and not moving, he or she may be unconscious. Unconsciousness is a life-threatening emergency. If the person does not respond to you in any way, assume he or she is unconscious. Make sure that someone calls 9-1-1 or the local emergency number right away.

Look for other signals of life-threatening injuries or injuries that may become life threatening. These include no breathing or trouble breathing, no signs of life or severe bleeding.

While you are checking the person, use your senses of sight, smell and hearing. They will help you notice anything abnormal. For example, you may notice an unusual smell that could be caused by a poison. You may see a bruise or a twisted arm or leg. You may hear the person say something that explains how he or she was injured.

Children and the Elderly

Keep in mind that it is often helpful to take a slightly different approach when you check and care for infants, children and elderly people in an emergency situation. For more information on checking and caring for infants, children, the elderly and others with special needs, see Chapter 12.

CALL

Calling for help is often the most important action you can take to help an ill or injured person. It will start emergency medical help on its way as fast as possible (Fig. 2-3).

When calling 9-1-1 or the local emergency number, provide the information that the call taker requests, including the location of the emergency and a description of the person's condition. *Do not* hang up before the dispatcher does. You might cut off

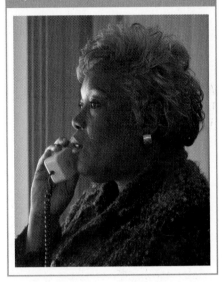

FIGURE 2-3 Calling for help is often the most important action you can take to help an ill or injured person.

some information the dispatcher needs. Whenever possible, ask a bystander to make the call for you.

Call First or *Care First?*

If you are the **only person at the scene**, you should first shout for help. If no one arrives, you will have to decide whether to *Call First* or *Care First*. In *Call First* situations, you would call 9-1-1 or the local emergency number before giving care. In *Care First* situations, you would give 2 minutes of care first and then call.

You should always *Call First* for—
- An unconscious adult or adolescent (age 12 years or older).
- A witnessed sudden collapse of a child or infant.
- An unconscious infant or child known to be at high risk for heart problems.

Call First situations are likely to be cardiac emergencies, such as sudden cardiac arrest or a witnessed sudden collapse of a child, in which time is critical. Research shows that the shorter the time from when a person

IDENTIFYING LIFE-THREATENING CONDITIONS

At times, you may be unsure if EMS personnel are needed. Your first aid training will help you make this decision. As a general rule, call 9-1-1 or the local emergency number if the person—

- Is or becomes unconscious.
- Has trouble breathing or is breathing in a strange way.
- Has chest discomfort, pain or pressure that persists for more than 3 to 5 minutes or that goes away and comes back.
- Is bleeding severely.
- Has a severe (critical) burn.
- Has pressure or pain in the abdomen that does not go away.
- Is vomiting blood or passing blood.
- Has a seizure that lasts more than 5 minutes or has multiple seizures.
- Has a seizure and is pregnant.
- Has a seizure and is diabetic.
- Fails to regain consciousness after a seizure.
- Has a sudden severe headache or slurred speech.
- Appears to have been poisoned.
- Has injuries to the head, neck or back.
- Has possible broken bones.

Also call for any of these situations:

- Fire or explosion
- Downed electrical wires
- Swiftly moving or rapidly rising water
- Presence of poisonous gas
- Motor vehicle collisions
- People who cannot be moved easily

The most important step you can take for a person who is unconscious or has some other life-threatening condition is to call for emergency medical help (Fig. 2-4).

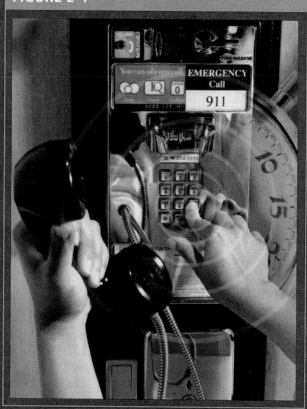

FIGURE 2-4

Make the call quickly and return to the person. If possible, send someone else to make the call.

With a life-threatening condition, the survival of a person often depends on both emergency medical help and the care you can give. You will have to use your best judgment, based on knowledge of your surroundings, information gained from this course and other training you may have received, to make the decision to call. It is often a good idea to ask a bystander to make the call while you give care.

WHAT HAPPENS WHEN YOU CALL 9-1-1

When your call is answered, you will be talking to an emergency call taker (or dispatcher) who is specially trained in dealing with crises over the phone (Fig. 2-5). The call taker will ask for your phone number and address and will ask other key questions to determine whether you need police, fire or medical assistance.

It may seem that the call taker asks a lot of questions. Focus on remaining calm so that you can give clear answers. The information you give will help the call taker send appropriate help, based on the severity of the emergency.

Once EMS is on the way, the call taker may stay on the line and continue to talk with you. Many call takers are also trained to give first aid instructions so they can assist you with life-saving techniques, such as cardiopulmonary resuscitation (CPR), rescue breathing or the use of an AED, until EMS arrives.

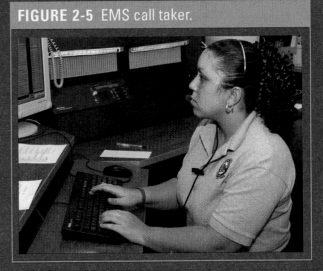

FIGURE 2-5 EMS call taker.

collapses to when CPR is initiated and he or she is given the first shock with an automated external defibrillator (AED), the greater the chance of survival for an adult or child 1 year old or older. For an infant or child with a known risk for heart problems, early access to the emergency medical services (EMS) system and the emergency medical care that results increases the chance of survival.

You should *Care First* for—

- An unwitnessed collapse of an unconscious person younger than 12 years old.
- Any victim of a drowning.

In *Care First* situations the conditions are often related to breathing emergencies, rather than sudden cardiac arrest. In these situations, provide support for airway, breathing and circulation (ABCs) through rescue breaths or chest compressions as appropriate. You will learn more about breathing emergencies in Chapter 4.

When making the call, find the nearest telephone as quickly as possible and immediately go back to the ill or injured person. Recheck the person for life-threatening conditions and give the necessary care.

CARE

Once you have checked the scene and the person and made a decision about calling 9-1-1, you may need to give care until EMS personnel arrive. To do so, follow these general guidelines:

- Do no further harm.
- Monitor the person's breathing and consciousness.
- Help the person rest in the most comfortable position.
- Keep the person from getting chilled or overheated.
- Reassure the person.
- Give any specific care needed.

WHEN TO CALL 9-1-1

If you came across any of the conditions below, would you know what to do? In emergencies involving more than one victim, it is important to be able to distinguish between life-threatening and nonlife-threatening conditions to know who needs care first. Place a checkmark in the box next to any life-threatening conditions for which 9-1-1 or the local emergency number should be called.

- ☐ Minor bruise on the arm
- ☐ Cat scratch on the cheek
- ☑ No signs of life
- ☒ No breathing
- ☐ Deep burn on the face
- ☒ Unconsciousness
- ☑ Trouble breathing
- ☐ Abrasion on the elbow
- ☐ Cut lip
- ☑ Persistent chest pain
- ☒ Severe bleeding that does not stop
- ☐ Mild sunburn on the shoulders
- ☐ Cramp in the thigh
- ☐ Pain in the abdomen that does not go away
- ☐ Vomiting blood
- ☐ Seizures
- ☐ Injury to the head
- ☐ Apparent poisoning
- ☐ Splinter in the finger
- ☐ Injured arm with bone showing through the skin
- ☐ Bloody nose

Transporting the Person Yourself

In some cases, you may decide to take the ill or injured person to a medical facility yourself instead of waiting for EMS personnel. If you plan to do so, ask someone to come with you to keep the person comfortable. Also, be sure you know the quickest route to the nearest medical facility capable of handling emergency care. Pay close attention to the ill or injured person and watch for any changes in his or her condition.

Never transport a person—
- When the trip may aggravate the injury or illness or cause additional injury.
- When the person has or may develop a life-threatening condition.
- If you are unsure of the nature of the injury or illness.

Calling for help is often the most important step you can take to help an ill or injured person.

If there is a life-threatening condition or a possibility of further injury, call 9-1-1 or the local emergency number and wait for help.

Discourage an ill or injured person from driving him- or herself to the hospital. An injury may restrict movement, or the victim may become groggy or faint. A sudden onset of pain may be distracting. Any of these conditions can make driving dangerous for the person, passengers, other drivers and pedestrians.

REACHING AND MOVING AN ILL OR INJURED PERSON: DO NO FURTHER HARM

One of the most dangerous threats to a seriously ill or injured person is unnecessary movement. Moving an injured person can cause additional injury and pain and complicate his or her recovery. Generally, you should not move an ill or injured person while giving care. However, in the following three situations, it would be appropriate:

- **When you are faced with immediate danger,** such as fire, lack of oxygen, risk of explosion or a collapsing structure.
- **When you have to get to another person who may have a more serious problem.** In this case, you may have to move a person with minor injuries to reach someone needing immediate care.
- **When it is necessary to give proper care.** For example, if someone needed CPR, he or she might have to be moved because CPR needs to be performed on a firm, level surface. If the surface or space is not adequate to give care, the person should be moved.

Once you decide to move an ill or injured person, you must quickly decide how to do so. Carefully consider your safety and the safety of the person. Base your decision on the dangers you are facing, the size and condition of the person, your abilities and condition and whether you have any help.

To improve your chances of successfully moving an ill or injured per-

WIRELESS 9-1-1: HUNDREDS OF MILLIONS SERVED

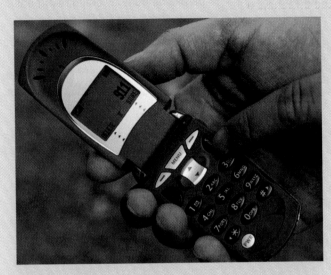

The 9-1-1 service was created in the United States in 1968 as a nationwide telephone number for the public to use to report emergencies and request emergency assistance. It gives the public direct access to an emergency communication center called a Public Service Answering Point, which is responsible for taking the appropriate action.

The numbers 9-1-1 were chosen because they best fit the needs of the public and the telephone companies. They are easy to remember and dial, and they have never been used as an office, area or service code. Today, an estimated 200 million people call 9-1-1 each year. At least 99 percent of the population and 96 percent of the geographic United States is covered by some type of 9-1-1 service.

According to the Federal Communications Commissions (FCC), over 50 million people now use wireless phones to call 9-1-1. That is more than double the number who used wireless phones to activate EMS in 1995. However, because wireless phones are not associated with one fixed location or address, it can be difficult for call takers to accurately determine the location of the caller or the emergency.

To help the call taker find your location if you call 9-1-1 on a wireless phone, it is important to remember the following tips:

- Tell the call taker the location of the emergency right away.
- Give the call taker your wireless phone number so that he or she can call you back if the call gets disconnected. This is especially important if you do not have a contract for service with a wireless service provider, because in these cases the call taker will have no way of obtaining your wireless phone number and will not be able to contact you.
- Learn to use the designated number in your state for highway accidents or other nonlife-threatening incidents. States often reserve specific numbers for these types of incidents. For example, "#77" is the number used for highway accidents in Virginia. The number to call for nonlife-threatening incidents in your state may be located in the front of your phone book.
- Do not program your phone to automatically dial 9-1-1 when one button, such as the "9" key, is pressed. Wireless 9-1-1 calls often occur when autodial keys are pressed unintentionally. This causes problems for emergency service call centers.
- If your wireless phone came pre-programmed with the autodial 9-1-1 feature already turned on, turn this feature off. Check your user manual to find out how.
- Lock your keypad when you are not using your wireless phone. This action also prevents accidental calls to 9-1-1.

SOURCES:
DISPATCH Monthly Magazine, www.911.dispatch.com. Accessed 6/24/04.
Federal Communications Commission, www.fcc.gov/911/enhanced. Accessed 6/24/04.
National Emergency Number Association, www.nena.org. Accessed 6/24/04.

son without injuring yourself or the person—

- Use your legs, not your back, when you bend.
- Bend at the knees and hips and avoid twisting your body.
- Walk forward when possible, taking small steps and looking where you are going.

- Avoid twisting or bending anyone with a possible head, neck or back injury.
- Do not move a person who is too large to move comfortably.

Emergency Moves

You can move a person to safety in many different ways, but no single way is best for every situation. The objective is to move the person without injuring yourself or causing further injury to the person. The following common types of emergency moves can all be done by one or two people and without any equipment.

Walking Assist. The most basic emergency move is the walking assist. Either one or two responders can use this method with a conscious person.

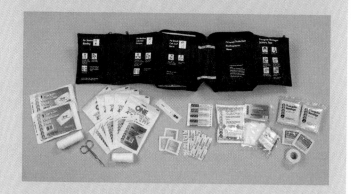

To perform a walking assist, place the ill or injured person's arm across your shoulders and hold it in place with one hand. Support the person with your other hand around the person's waist (Fig. 2-6, A). In this way, your body acts as a crutch, supporting the person's weight while you both walk. A second responder, if present, can support the person in the same way on the other side (Fig. 2-6, B). Do not use this assist if you suspect that the person has a head, neck or back injury.

Pack-Strap Carry. The pack-strap carry can be used with conscious and unconscious people. Using it with an unconscious person requires a second responder to help position the

FIGURE 2-6, A-B In a walking assist, your body acts as a crutch, supporting the person's weight while you both walk.

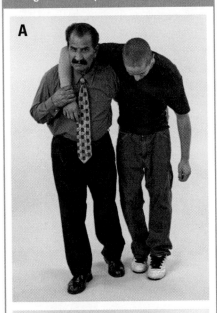

A

B

FIRST AID CHALLENGE

You have learned the emergency action steps: CHECK—CALL—CARE. Would you know what to do in an emergency? When there is more than one person who needs care, would you know which one to care for first? Test your knowledge of the emergency action steps by deciding what you would do in each of the four situations below.

1. Two girls were playing with a ball and fell down the stairs. One girl is holding her forehead and appears to be conscious. The other girl is face-down and appears to be unconscious (Fig. 2-7).
2. The little girl is sitting up, conscious and holding her knee. The little boy is laying with his leg entangled, he appears to be unconscious (Fig. 2-8).
3. The boy is sitting on the bridge and appears to be conscious and warming his hands by blowing on them. The girl appears to be laying down and experiencing signals of hypothermia (Fig. 2-9).
4. A 10-year-old child darts onto the road between two parked cars and is struck by an oncoming bicyclist. Both people are injured on the busy road. The bicyclist is conscious and holding her arm. The 10-year-old child is quiet and not moving. (Fig. 2-10).

FIGURE 2-7

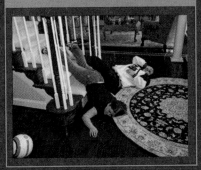

FIGURE 2-8

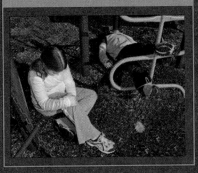

FIGURE 2-9

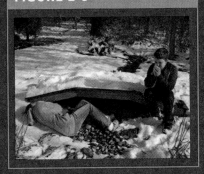

FIGURE 2-10

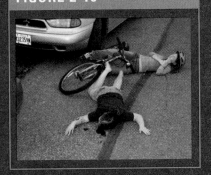

FIGURE 2-11, A-B The pack-strap carry.

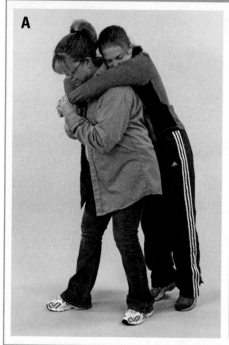

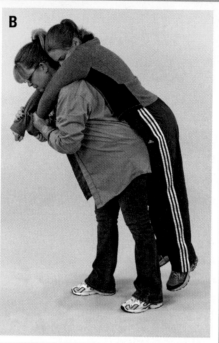

FIGURE 2-12, A-C The two-person seat carry.

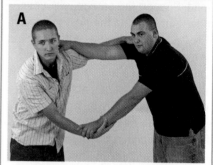

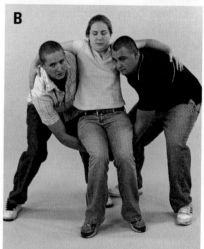

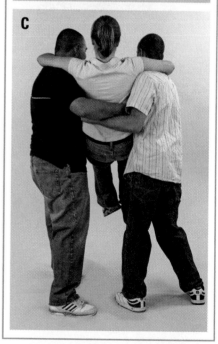

ill or injured person on your back. To perform the pack-strap carry, have the person stand or have a second responder support the person. Position yourself with your back to the person, back straight, knees bent, so that your shoulders fit into the person's armpits (Fig. 2-11, A). Cross the person's arms in front of you and grasp the person's wrists. Lean forward slightly and pull the person up and onto your back. Stand up and walk to safety (Fig. 2-11, B). Depending on the size of the person, you may be able to hold both of his or her wrists with one hand, leaving your other hand free to help maintain balance, open doors and remove obstructions. Do not use this assist if you suspect that the person has a head, neck or back injury.

Two-Person Seat Carry. The two-person seat carry requires a second responder. This carry can be used for any person who is conscious and not seriously injured. Put one arm behind the person's thighs and the other across the person's back. Interlock your arms with those of a second responder behind the person's legs and across his or her back (Fig. 2-12, A). Lift the person in the "seat" formed by the responders' arms (Fig. 2-12, B-C).

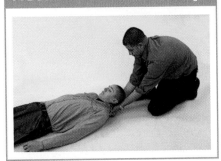

FIGURE 2-13 The clothes drag.

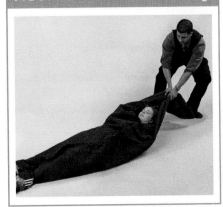

FIGURE 2-14 The blanket drag.

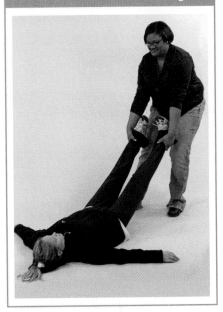

FIGURE 2-15 The foot drag.

Clothes Drag. The clothes drag can be used to move a conscious or unconscious person suspected of having a head, neck or back injury. This move helps keep the person's head, neck and back stabilized. Grasp the person's clothing behind the neck, gathering enough to secure a firm grip. Using the clothing, pull the person (head-first) to safety (Fig. 2-13).

During this move, the person's head is cradled by clothing and the responder's arms. Be aware that this move is exhausting and may cause back strain for the responder, even when done properly.

Blanket Drag. The blanket drag can be used to move a person in an emergency situation when equipment is limited. Keep the person between you and the blanket. Gather half the blanket and place it against the person's side. Roll the person as a unit toward you. Reach over and place the blanket so that it will be positioned under the person, then roll the person onto the blanket. Gather the blanket at the head and move the person (Fig. 2-14).

Foot Drag. Use the foot drag to move a person who is too large to carry or move in any other way. Firmly grasp the person's ankles and move backward. Pull the person in a straight line, and be careful not to bump the person's head (Fig. 2-15).

DEVELOPING A PLAN OF ACTION

Emergencies can happen quickly. There may not be time to think about what to do. There may only be time to react. You can improve your response and the outcome of emergencies by developing an emergency plan.

A good plan identifies the emergencies you are most likely to face, the possible locations and people involved. It also establishes the steps you would take in the emergencies, as well as prevention strategies.

The first step in putting together an emergency plan is to gather information. Here are some suggestions on where to start.

Think about your home.

- Style of home (e.g., mobile, high-rise, duplex, single family)
- Type of construction (e.g., wood, brick)
- Location of sleeping areas (e.g., basement, ground floor, second floor)
- Location of windows
- Number and location of smoke alarms
- Location of gasoline, solvent or paint storage
- Number and types of locks on doors
- Location of telephones
- Location of flashlights
- Location of fire extinguisher
- Location of first aid kit

Think about who lives there.

- Number of people
- Number of people over 65 or under 6 years of age
- Number of people sleeping above or below the ground floor
- Number of people unable to exit without help

Think about the types of emergencies that you may face.

- Injuries (e.g., fall or cut)
- Illnesses (e.g., stroke or heart attack)
- Natural disasters (e.g., tornado or earthquake)
- Fire

Now get some help from the people you live with. Write down the list of emergencies and under each one list—

1. How the emergency would affect your home.
2. How you would like the people in your home to react.
3. The steps you have already taken to prevent or minimize the effect of the emergency.
4. The steps you still need to take.

You can get more help from the following sources:

- Insurance companies
- Your city or county emergency management office
- Your police department
- Your fire department/rescue squad

Try to imagine as many situations as possible for each emergency. Think about emergencies away from home. Use the same process to decide what to do.

When you reach a decision, write it down. You now have a personal emergency plan. Practice it. Keep it current.

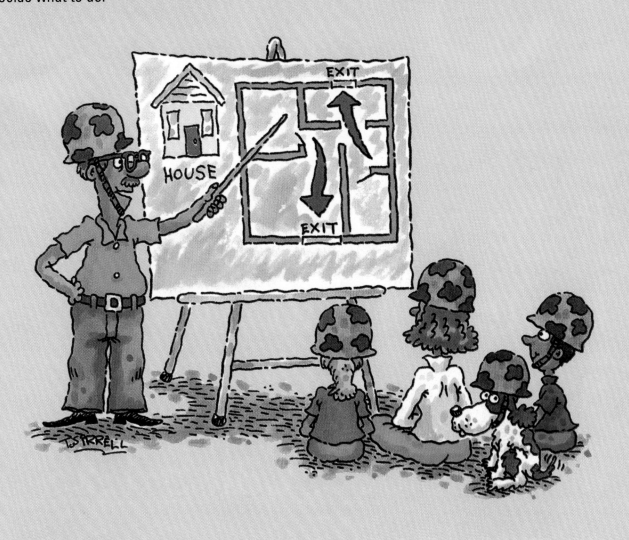

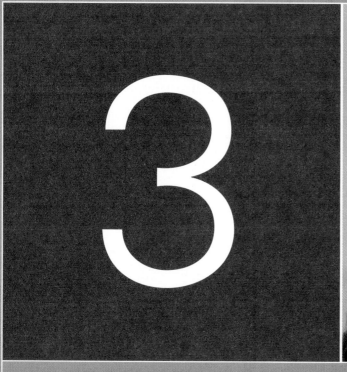

3

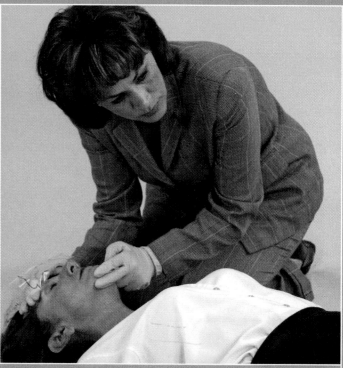

If the person does not respond to you, assume he or she is unconscious. Call 9-1-1 or the local emergency number at once!

Chapter 3

Checking an Ill or Injured Person

When you reach an ill or injured person, check first for life-threatening conditions such as unconsciousness. In many emergencies this will be obvious but in some situations you may not be able to tell.

If you are not sure whether someone is unconscious, tap him or her on the shoulder and ask if he or she is okay. Use the person's name if you know it. Speak loudly. If you are not sure whether an infant is unconscious, check by flicking the bottom of the infant's foot and/or tapping the infant's shoulders and shout to see if the infant responds (Fig. 3-1).

If the person does not respond to you, assume that he or she is unconscious. Have someone call 9-1-1 or the local emergency number.

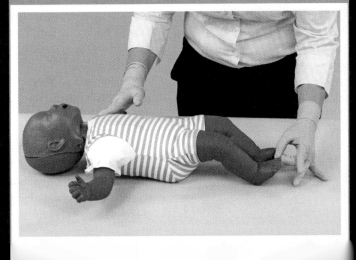

FIGURE 3-1 Checking an unconscious infant.

CHECKING A CONSCIOUS PERSON

For purposes of first aid, an adult is defined as someone about age 12 or older; someone between the ages of 1 and 12 (school age) is considered a child; and an infant is someone less than 1 year old. When using pediatric AED equipment, a child is someone between the ages of 1 and 8 or weighing less than 55 pounds.

If you determine that an ill or injured person is conscious and has no immediate life-threatening conditions, you can begin to check for other conditions that may need care. Checking a conscious person with no immediate life-threatening conditions involves two basic steps—

- Interview the person and bystanders.
- Check the person from head to toe.

Conducting Interviews

Ask the person and bystanders simple questions to learn more about what happened. Keep these interviews brief (Fig. 3-2). Remember to first identify yourself and to get the person's consent to give care. Begin by asking the person's name. This will make him or her feel more comfortable. Gather additional information by asking the person the following questions:

- What happened?
- Do you feel pain or discomfort anywhere?
- Do you have any allergies?
- Do you have any medical conditions or are you taking any medication?

If the person feels pain, ask him or her to describe it and to tell you where it is located. Descriptions will often include terms such as burning, crushing, throbbing, aching or sharp pain. Ask when the pain started and what the person was doing when it began. Ask the person to rate his or her pain on a scale of 1 to 10 (1 being mild and 10 being severe).

Sometimes an ill or injured person will not be able to give you the information that you need. Infants or children may be frightened, or the person may not speak your language. Remember to question family members, friends or bystanders as well. They may be able to give you helpful information or help you communicate with the person. You will learn more about communicating with people with special needs in Chapter 12.

Write down the information you learn during the interviews or, preferably, have someone else write it down for you. Be sure to give the information to emergency medical services (EMS) personnel when they arrive. It may help them to determine the type of medical care the person should receive.

Next you will need to thoroughly check the ill or injured person so that you do not overlook any problems. For adults, check from head to toe. For infants and children, check from toe to head. This will be less emotionally threatening. It is often helpful to check a young child while he or she is seated in his or her parent or guardian's lap.

Checking from Head to Toe

When checking a conscious person—

- Do not move areas in which they have discomfort or if you suspect head, neck or back injury.
- Check the person's head by examining the scalp, face, ears, nose and mouth.
- Look for cuts, bruises, bumps or depressions. Think of how the body usually looks. If you are unsure if a body part or limb looks injured, check it against the opposite limb or the other side of the body.
- Watch for changes in consciousness. Notice if the person is drowsy, not alert or confused.
- Look for changes in the person's breathing. A healthy person breathes normally, quietly and easily. Infants and young children generally breathe faster than adults. Breathing that is not normal includes noisy breathing, such as gasping for air; rasping, gurgling or whistling sounds; breathing that is unusually fast or slow; and breathing that is painful.

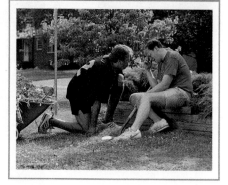

FIGURE 3-2 Ask simple questions and keep interviews brief.

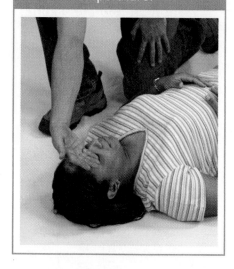

FIGURE 3-3 Feel the skin with the back of your hand to determine its temperature.

- Notice how the skin looks and feels. Skin can provide clues that a person is ill or injured. Feel the person's forehead with the back of your hand to determine if the skin feels unusually damp, dry, cool or hot (Fig. 3-3). Note if it is red, pale or ashen.
- Look over the body. Ask again about any areas that hurt. Ask the person to move each part of the body that does not hurt. Ask the person to gently move his or her head from side to side (Fig. 3-4). Check the shoulders by asking the person to shrug them (Fig. 3-5). Check the chest and abdomen by asking the person to take a deep breath (Fig. 3-6). Ask the person to move his or her fingers, hands and arms (Fig. 3-7). Check the hips and legs in the same way (Fig. 3-8). *During a head-to-toe check, ask the person not to move any parts that hurt.* Watch the person's face and listen for signals of discomfort or pain as you check for injuries.

WATCH FACE + LISTEN FOR SIGNALS OF DISCOMFORT

FIGURE 3-5 Ask the person to shrug his or her shoulders to check the shoulders.

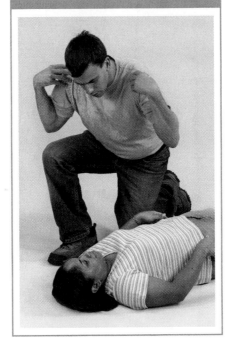

FIGURE 3-6 To check the chest and abdomen, ask the person to breathe deeply and then blow the air out.

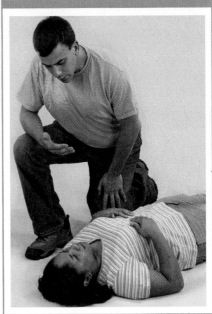

FIGURE 3-4 Ask the person to gently move his or her head from side to side to check the neck.

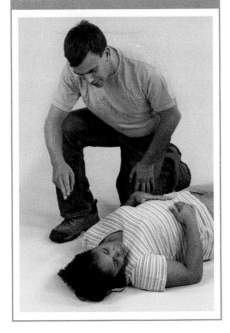

FIGURE 3-7 Ask the person to move his or her fingers, hands and arms.

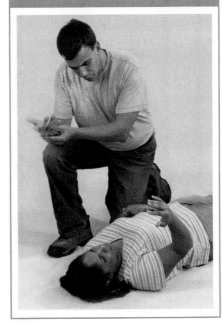

FIGURE 3-8 Ask the person to bend his or her legs.

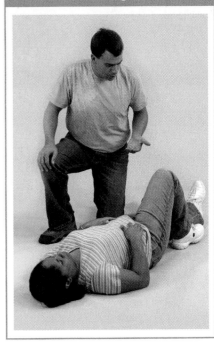

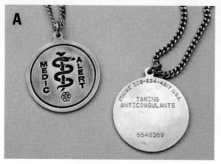
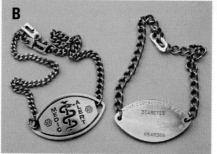

Medic Alert is a Federally Registered Trademark and Service Mark © 2006. All rights reserved.

- Look for a medical ID tag (Fig. 3-9, A) or bracelet (Fig. 3-9, B) on the person's wrist, neck or ankle. A tag will give you medical information about the person, explain how to care for certain conditions and list whom to call for help.

When you have finished checking, determine if the person can move his or her body without any pain. If the person can, and there are no other signals of injury, have him or her attempt to rest in a sitting or other comfortable position (Fig. 3-10). When the person feels ready, help him or her stand up (Fig. 3-11). Determine what additional care is needed and whether to call 9-1-1 or the local emergency number.

As you continue reading you will learn more about life-threatening situations, such as breathing and cardiac emergencies.

FIGURE 3-10 If there are no signals of obvious injuries, help the person into a comfortable position.

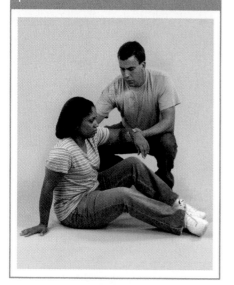

FIGURE 3-11 Help the person to slowly stand when he or she is ready.

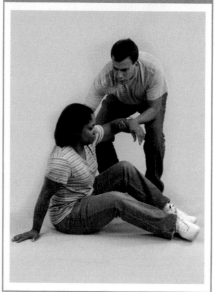

CHECKING AN UNCONSCIOUS PERSON

If you find that the person is unconscious and 9-1-1 or the local emergency number has been called, find out if there are other conditions that threaten the person's life. Always check to see if an unconscious person—

- Has an open airway.
- Shows signs of life (movement or breathing).
- Is bleeding severely.

An easy way to remember what you need to check is to think of ABC, which stands for—

- Airway—open the airway.
- Breathing—check for movement or breathing.
- Circulation—check for signs of life (including a pulse for a child or infant) and severe bleeding.

Airway

Once you or someone else has called 9-1-1 or the local emergency number, you must check to see if the person has an open airway and is breathing. An open airway allows air to enter the lungs for the person to breathe. If the airway is blocked, the person cannot breathe. This is a life-threatening condition.

When someone is unconscious and lying on his or her back, the tongue may fall to the back of the throat and block the airway. To open an unconscious person's airway, push down on his or her forehead while pulling up on the bony part of the jaw with two or three fingers of your other hand to lift the chin (Fig. 3-13). This procedure, known as the *head-tilt/chin-lift technique*, moves the tongue away from the back of the throat, allowing air to enter the lungs.

Breathing

After opening the airway, you must check an unconscious person carefully for signals of breathing. Look, listen and feel for these signals.

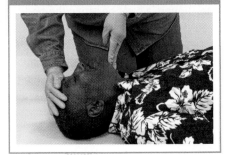

FIGURE 3-13 Open an unconscious person's airway using the head-tilt/chin-lift technique.

CHECKING FOR A PULSE—CHILD AND INFANT

To find out if a child's or infant's heart is beating, check for a pulse (Fig. 3-12, A-B) for no more than 10 seconds.

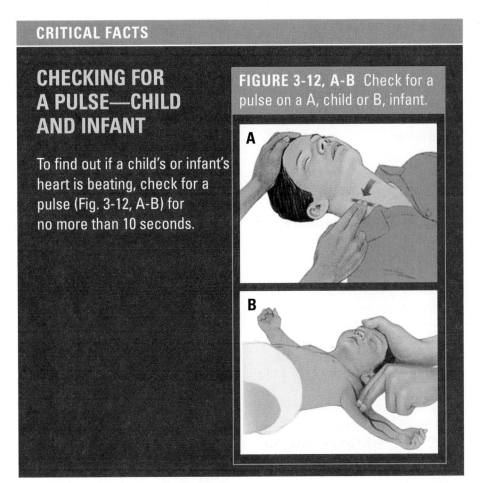

FIGURE 3-12, A-B Check for a pulse on a A, child or B, infant.

Position yourself so that you can hear and feel air as it escapes from the nose and mouth. At the same time, look to see if the victim's chest clearly rises and falls. Look, listen and feel for movement and breathing for no more than 10 seconds (Fig. 3-14). If the person is not breathing, give 2 rescue breaths with each breath lasting 1 second (Fig. 3-15). If the air goes in (chest clearly rises) check for severe bleeding and pulse for children and infants.

In an unconscious adult you may detect an irregular, gasping or shallow breath. This is known as an agonal breath. Do not confuse this with normal breathing. You should begin CPR immediately. Agonal breaths do not occur frequently in children.

Sometimes food, liquid or other objects will block the person's airway. When this happens, you will need to remove whatever is blocking the airway. You will learn how to recognize and give care for an obstructed airway in Chapter 4.

If air does go in but the person is not breathing, you will need to perform rescue breathing for infants and children. Rescue breathing is a technique used to provide a nonbreathing victim with oxygen. You will learn how to perform rescue breathing in Chapter 4.

FIGURE 3-14 Look, listen and feel for movement and breathing for no more than 10 seconds.

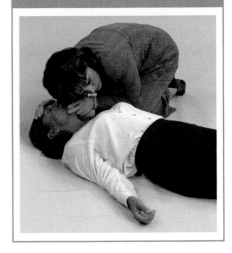

FIGURE 3-15 Keep the airway open and give 2 rescue breaths.

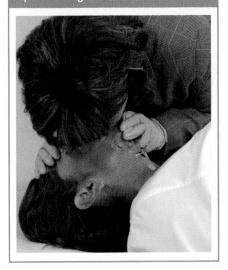

If the person is breathing, his or her heart is beating and is circulating blood. In this case, maintain an open airway by using the head-tilt/chin-lift technique as you continue to look for other life-threatening conditions.

Circulation

It is very important to recognize breathing emergencies in children and infants, and to act before the heart stops beating. Adults' hearts frequently stop beating because they are diseased. Infants' and children's hearts, however, are usually healthy. When an infant or child's heart stops, it is usually the result of a breathing emergency.

If an adult is not breathing and you have given him or her 2 rescue breaths, you must then assume the problem is a cardiac emergency and begin CPR immediately.

If a child or infant shows no signs of life (movement or breathing), you will have to check for a pulse for no more than 10 seconds (see Fig. 3-12, A-B). If you find a pulse but no breathing, give rescue breathing. If the child or infant does not show signs of life or a pulse, the heart is not beating properly. You must keep blood circulating in the child's or infant's body until emergency medical help arrives. To do this, you will have to perform cardiopulmonary resuscitation (CPR). Rescue breathing is discussed in Chapter 4. CPR is discussed in Chapter 5.

Severe Bleeding

Check for severe bleeding by looking over the person's body from head to toe for signals such as blood-soaked clothing or blood spurting out of a wound (Fig. 3-16). Bleeding usually looks worse than it is. A small amount of blood on a slick surface or mixed with water almost always looks like a

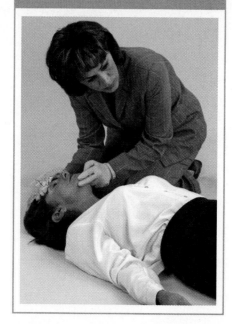

FIGURE 3-16 Check for severe bleeding by scanning from head to toe.

great deal of blood. It is not always easy to recognize severe bleeding.

SHOCK

When the body is healthy, three conditions are needed to keep the right amount of blood flowing—

- The heart must be working well.
- An adequate amount of oxygen-rich blood must be circulating in the body.
- The blood vessels must be intact and able to adjust blood flow.

Shock is a condition in which the circulatory system fails to deliver oxygen-rich blood to the body's tissues and vital organs. When the body's organs, such as the brain, heart and lungs, do not receive this blood, they fail to function properly. This triggers a series of responses that produce specific signals known as shock. These responses are the body's attempt to maintain adequate blood flow.

When someone is injured or becomes suddenly ill, these normal body functions may be interrupted. In cases of minor injury or illness, this interruption is brief because the body is able to compensate quickly. With more severe injuries or illnesses, however, the body may be unable to adjust. When the body is unable to meet its demand for oxygen because blood fails to circulate adequately, shock occurs.

Signals of Shock

The signals that indicate a person may be going into shock include—
- Restlessness or irritability.
- Altered level of consciousness.
- Nausea or vomiting.
- Pale, ashen, cool, moist skin.
- Rapid breathing and pulse.
- Excessive thirst.

Caring for Shock

Caring for shock involves the following simple steps:
- **Call 9-1-1 or the local emergency number immediately.** Shock cannot be managed effectively by first aid alone. A person suffering from shock requires emergency medical care as soon as possible.
- **Have the person lie down.** This is often the most comfortable position (Fig. 3-17, A). Helping the person rest comfortably is important because pain can intensify the body's stress and speed up the progression of shock. Helping the person rest in a more comfortable position may lessen any pain.
- **Control any external bleeding.**
  - Elevate the person's legs about 12 inches, unless you suspect head, neck or back injuries or possible broken bones involving the hips or legs (Fig. 3-17, B). If you are unsure of the person's condition, leave him or her lying flat.

FIGURE 3-17, A-C A, Help a victim of shock lie down. B, Elevate the person's legs about 12 inches. C, Keep the person from getting chilled or overheated.

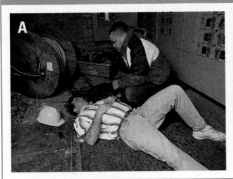
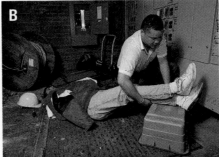
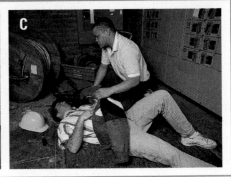

- Help the person maintain normal body temperature (Fig. 3-17, C). If the person is cool, try to cover him or her to avoid chilling.
- Do not give the person anything to eat or drink, even though he or she is likely to be thirsty. The person's condition may be severe enough to require surgery, in which case it is better if the stomach is empty.
- Reassure the person.
- Continue to monitor the person's airway, breathing and circulation.

Checking a Conscious Person

STEP 1
CHECK scene, then **CHECK** person.

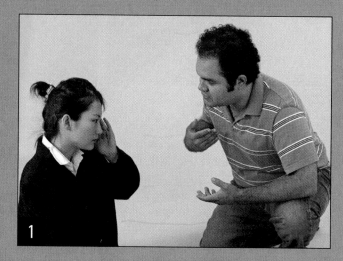

STEP 2
Obtain consent.

STEP 3
CALL 9-1-1 for any life-threatening conditions.

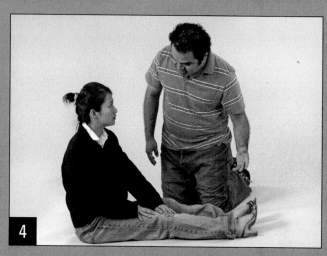

STEP 4
Ask the person—

- What is your name?
- What happened?
- Where do you feel pain or discomfort?
- Do you have any allergies?
- Do you have any medical conditions?
- Are you taking any medications?
- When did you last eat or drink anything?

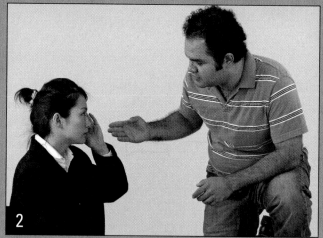

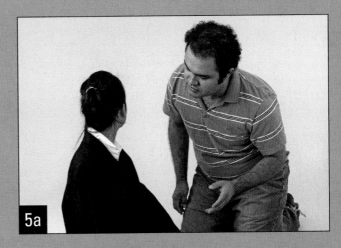

STEP 5

CHECK head to toe for—

- Bleeding, fluids or wounds.
- Skin color and temperature.
- Medical ID bracelets and necklaces.
- Observable signals of pain.

(**TIP:** For infants and children, check from toe to head. Do not separate them from parent or guardian.)

CHILD TOE TO HEAD

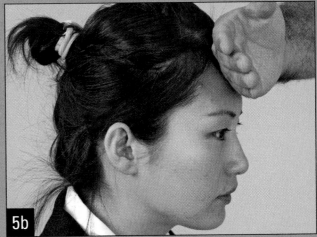

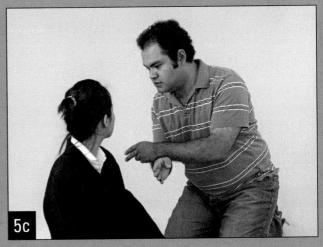

(CONSCIOUS PERSON)

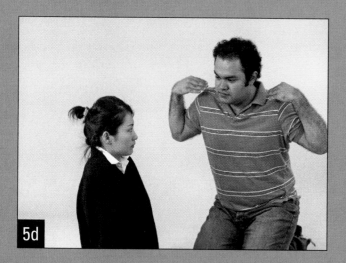

5d

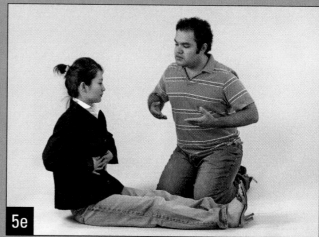

5e

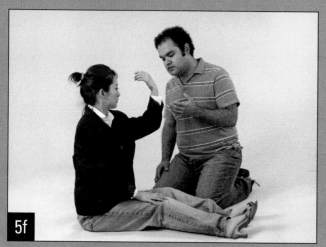

5f

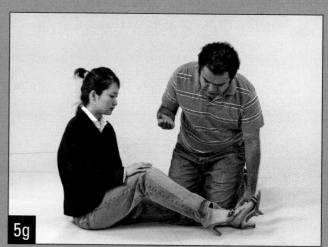

5g

STEP 6

Continue to monitor Airway, Breathing and
Circulation (**ABCs**).

Checking an Unconscious Adult

(APPEARS TO BE UNCONSCIOUS)

FOR ADULT (AGE 12 OR OLDER)

*(**TIP:** Wear disposable gloves and personal protective equipment.)*

STEP 1
CHECK scene, then **CHECK** person.

STEP 2
Tap shoulder and shout, "Are you okay?"

STEP 3
No response, **CALL 9-1-1**.

*(**TIP:** If an unconscious person is face-down— Roll face-up supporting head, neck and back.)*

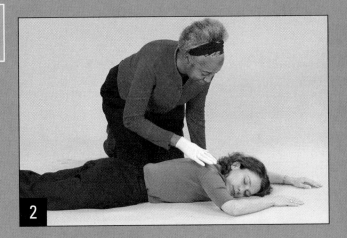

STEP 4
Open airway (tilt head, lift chin), **CHECK** for signs of life (movement and breathing) for no more than 10 seconds.

STEP 5
If no breathing, give 2 rescue breaths.

*(**TIP:** Irregular, gasping or shallow breaths are NOT effective.)*

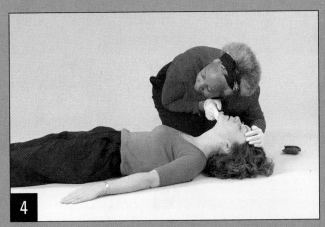

STEP 6
If breathing, place in recovery position and monitor Airway, Breathing and Circulation (**ABCs**).

WHAT TO DO NEXT
IF BREATHS GO IN—Quickly scan the body for severe bleeding and get into position to perform CPR or use an AED (if AED is immediately available).

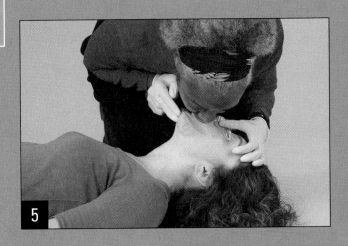

Checking an Unconscious Child

FOR CHILD (AGES 1 TO 12)

*(**TIP:** Wear disposable gloves and personal protective equipment.)*

STEP 1
CHECK scene, then **CHECK** child.

STEP 2
Obtain consent from parent or guardian, if present.

STEP 3
Tap shoulder and shout, "Are you okay?"

STEP 4
No response, **CALL 9-1-1**.

If alone—

- Give about **2** minutes of **CARE**.
- Then **CALL 9-1-1**.

*(**TIP:** If an unconscious child is face-down— Roll face-up supporting head, neck and back.)*

STEP 5
Open airway (tilt head, lift chin), **CHECK** for signs of life (movement and breathing) for no more than 10 seconds.

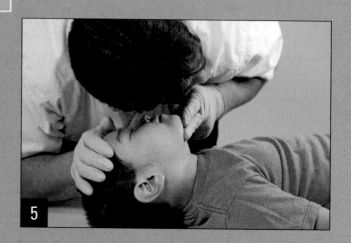

STEP 6

If no breathing, give **2** rescue breaths.

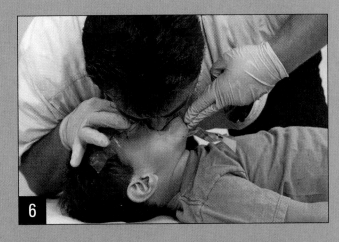

STEP 7

If breaths go in, **CHECK** for pulse (and severe bleeding).

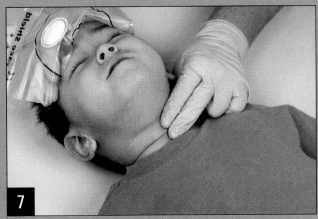

STEP 8

If breathing, place in recovery position and monitor **ABCs**.

WHAT TO DO NEXT

IF BREATHS DO NOT GO IN—Give care for unconscious choking.

IF PULSE, BUT NO BREATHING—Give rescue breathing.

OR

IF NO PULSE—give CPR or use an AED (if AED is immediately available).

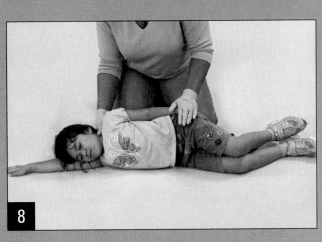

Checking an Unconscious Infant

FOR INFANT (UNDER AGE 1)

*(**TIP:** Wear disposable gloves and personal protective equipment.)*

STEP 1

CHECK scene, then **CHECK** infant.

STEP 2

Obtain consent from parent or guardian, if present.

STEP 3

Flick foot or tap shoulder and shout, "Are you okay?"

STEP 4

No response, **CALL 9-1-1**.

If alone—
- Give about **2** minutes of **CARE**.
- Then **CALL 9-1-1**.

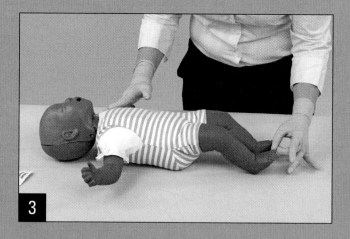

STEP 5

If an unconscious infant is face-down—
Roll face-up supporting head, neck and back.

STEP 6

Open airway (tilt head, lift chin), **CHECK** for signs of life (movement and breathing) for no more than 10 seconds.

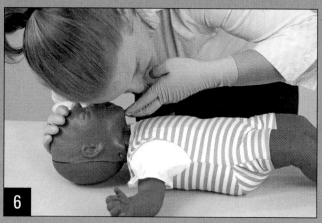

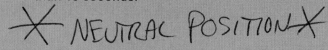

NEUTRAL POSITION

STEP 7

If no breathing, give **2** rescue breaths.

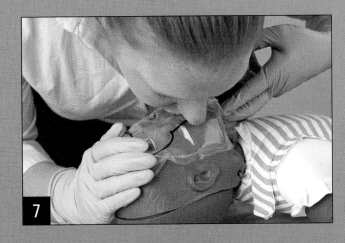

STEP 8

If breaths go in, **CHECK** for pulse (and severe bleeding).

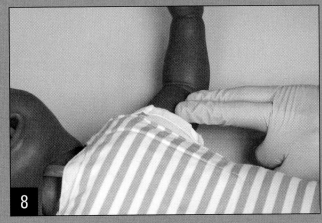

STEP 9

If breathing, place in recovery position and monitor **ABCs**.

WHAT TO DO NEXT

IF BREATHS DO NOT GO IN—
Give care for unconscious choking.

IF PULSE, BUT NO BREATHING—
Give rescue breathing

OR

IF NO PULSE—Give CPR.

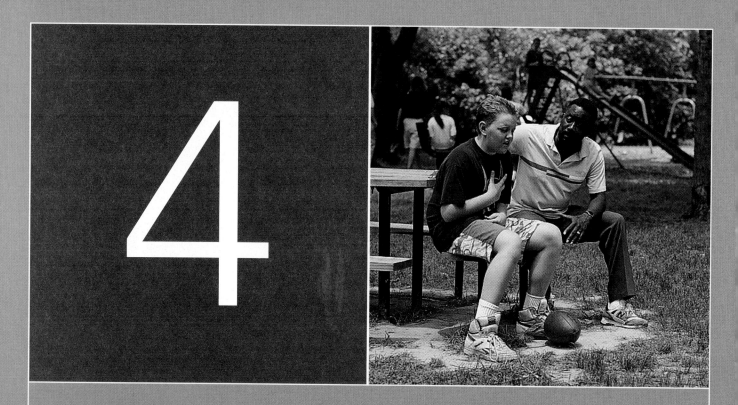

4

When a person is not breathing, call 9-1-1 or the local emergency number immediately!

Chapter 4

When Seconds Count

LIFE-THREATENING EMERGENCIES

In a life-threatening emergency you must help at once. It may only be a matter of seconds before the ill or injured person dies. An emergency is life threatening if the person is unconscious, not breathing, has trouble breathing, shows no signs of life or is bleeding severely.

Fortunately, most of the ill or injured people you are likely to encounter will be conscious. They probably will be able to indicate what is wrong by speaking or gesturing to you. You will be able to ask them questions. But if you are unable to communicate with a person, it can be difficult to know what is wrong.

Unconsciousness

As you learned in Chapter 3, if an ill or injured person is unconscious, a life-threatening emergency exists. In general, if you are alone and you find that a person is unconscious, you should *Call First*. This means you should call 9-1-1 or the local emergency number *before* giving care, and then return immediately to the ill or injured person. However, if someone else is available, have that person make the call while you continue to check to see if the person is breathing, shows signs of life or is bleeding severely.

If you are alone and the ill or injured person is a child or an infant who is not breathing and does not have a history of heart problems or whose collapse was unwitnessed, you will need to *Care First*. This means you should give care for about 2 minutes before calling 9-1-1. If the child is small enough, carry him or her with you to the phone while you continue to give rescue breaths. (You will learn more about giving rescue breaths and rescue breathing later in this chapter in the section called "Breathing Emergencies.") There is usually no need to move the person as long as he or she is breathing normally.

In some cases, the person may be unconscious but breathing normally and showing signs of life. If the person vomits, roll him or her onto one side and clear the mouth (Fig. 4-1). If the person stops breathing, place the person on his or her back and breathe for the person as described later in this manual. If you are alone and have to leave the person for any reason, such as to call for help, place the person in a recovery position. Figure 4-2, A, shows how to place a person without a suspected spinal injury in a recovery position. Figure 4-2, B, shows how to place a person with a suspected

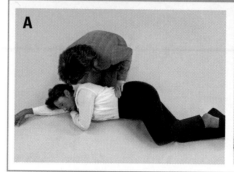
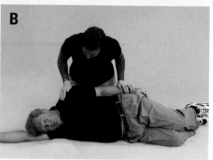

FIGURE 4-2, A-B A, Placing a person without a suspected spinal injury in a recovery position. B, Placing a person with a suspected spinal injury in a modified H.A.IN.E.S. recovery position.

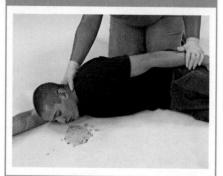

FIGURE 4-1 If the person vomits, roll him or her onto one side and clear the mouth.

spinal injury in a recovery position. Placing a person in a recovery position will help the airway remain open and clear if he or she vomits.

If the person has been in the recovery position for 30 minutes or more and begins to show signs of loss of circulation to the lower arm (such as pale, ashen or grayish skin that is cool to the touch), turn him or her to the opposite side.

If you suspect a head, neck or back injury and a clear, open airway can be maintained, do not move the person unnecessarily. If a clear airway **cannot** be maintained, or if you must leave the person to get help or to get an AED, move the person to his or her side while keeping the head, neck or back in a straight line by placing in a modified High Arm In Endangered Spine (H.A.IN.E.S.) position.

Breathing Emergencies

The human body needs a constant supply of oxygen to survive. When you breathe through your nose and mouth, air travels down your throat, through your windpipe and into your lungs. This pathway from the nose and mouth to the lungs is called the *airway*. As you might imagine, an infant or child's airway is much smaller than an adult's

airway. But for all human beings, the airway must be open in order for air to reach the lungs.

Once air reaches the lungs, oxygen in the air is transferred to the blood. The heart pumps the blood through the body. The blood flows through the blood vessels, taking the oxygen to the brain and heart, as well as to all other parts of the body.

A breathing emergency happens when air cannot travel freely and easily into the lungs. Some emergencies are life threatening because they greatly cut down on the oxygen the body receives or because they cut off the oxygen entirely. As a result, the heart soon stops beating and blood no longer moves through the body. Without oxygen, brain cells can begin to die in 4 to 6 minutes (Fig. 4-3). Unless the brain receives oxygen within minutes, permanent brain damage or death will result.

Respiratory Distress and Respiratory Arrest. A breathing problem so severe that it threatens a person's life is considered a breathing emergency. There are two types of breathing emergencies: *respiratory distress* and *respiratory arrest*. Respiratory distress is a condition in which breathing becomes

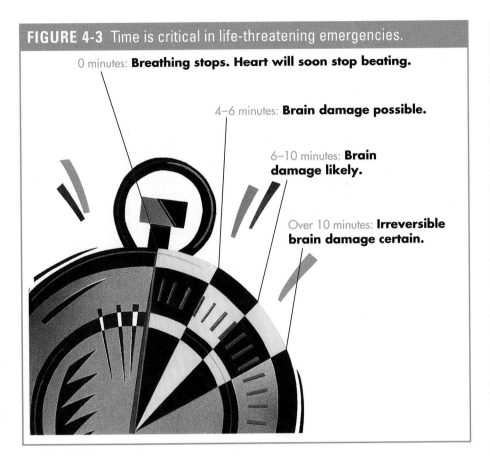

FIGURE 4-3 Time is critical in life-threatening emergencies.

0 minutes: **Breathing stops. Heart will soon stop beating.**

4–6 minutes: **Brain damage possible.**

6–10 minutes: **Brain damage likely.**

Over 10 minutes: **Irreversible brain damage certain.**

SIGNALS OF BREATHING EMERGENCIES

- Trouble breathing
  - Slow or rapid breathing
  - Unusually deep or shallow breathing
  - Gasping for breath
  - Wheezing, gurgling or making high-pitched noises
- Unusually moist or cool skin
- Flushed, pale, ashen or bluish skin color
- Shortness of breath
- Dizziness or lightheadedness
- Pain in the chest or tingling in hands, feet or lips
- Apprehensive or fearful feelings

difficult. It is the most common breathing emergency. Respiratory distress can lead to respiratory arrest, a condition in which breathing stops.

Respiratory distress can be caused by—

- A partially obstructed airway.
- Illness.
- Chronic conditions such as asthma.
- Electrocution.
- Heart attack.
- Injury to the head, chest, lungs or abdomen.
- Allergic reactions.
- Drugs.
- Poisoning.
- Emotional distress.

It is very important to recognize breathing emergencies in children and infants and to act before the heart stops beating. Adult hearts frequently stop beating because they are diseased. Infant and children's hearts, however, are usually healthy. When an infant or child's heart stops, it is usually the result of a breathing emergency.

No matter what the age of the person, trouble breathing can be the first signal of a more serious emergency such as a heart problem. Recognizing the signals of breathing problems and giving care are often the keys to preventing these problems from becoming more serious emergencies.

Trouble Breathing. Normal breathing is easy and quiet. A person does not appear to be working hard or struggling to breathe. The person is not making noise when breathing. Breaths are not fast or far apart and breathing does not cause discomfort or pain.

If you do encounter someone with a breathing problem, it will most likely be a conscious person who is having trouble breathing. You can usually identify a breathing problem by watching and listening to the person's breathing and by asking the person how he or she feels.

Although breathing problems have many causes, you do not need to know the exact cause of a breathing emergency to care for it. You do need to be able to recognize when a person is having trouble breathing or is not breathing at all.

Some Conditions that Cause Breathing Emergencies

Asthma

Asthma is a condition that narrows the air passages. An asthma attack happens when a trigger, such as exercise, cold air, allergens or other irritants, causes the airway to swell and narrow. This makes breathing difficult, which is frightening.

The Centers for Disease Control and Prevention (CDC) estimated that in 2003, nearly 30 million Americans were affected by asthma. Asthma is more common in children and young adults than in older adults, but its frequency and severity is increasing in all age groups in the United States. Asthma is the third-ranking cause of hospitalization among those younger than age 15.

You can often tell when a person is having an asthma attack by the hoarse whistling sound he or she makes while exhaling. This sound, known as wheezing, occurs because air becomes trapped in the lungs. Coughing after exercise, crying or laughing are other signals that an asthma attack is taking place. Usually, people diagnosed with asthma control their attacks with medication. These medications stop the muscle spasm that causes asthma and open the airway, which makes breathing easier.

For more information on asthma, see Chapter 13.

Emphysema

Emphysema is a disease that involves damage to the lungs' air sacs. It is a chronic (long-lasting or frequently recurring) disease that worsens over time. The most common signal of emphysema is shortness of breath. Exhaling is extremely difficult. In advanced cases, the affected person may feel restless, confused and weak, and may even go into respiratory or cardiac arrest.

Bronchitis

Bronchitis is a condition that causes the bronchial tubes to become swollen and irritated. This inflammation causes a buildup of mucus that blocks the passage of air and air exchange in the lungs. Chronic bronchitis is most commonly caused by long-term smoking but it can also be caused by exposure to irritants and pollutants in the environment. A person with bronchitis will typically have a persistent cough and may feel tightness in the chest and have trouble breathing. As with emphysema, the person may also feel restless, confused and weak, and may even go into respiratory or cardiac arrest.

Hyperventilation

Hyperventilation occurs when a person breathes faster and more shallowly than normal. When this happens, the body does not take in enough oxygen to meet its demands. People who are hyperventilating feel as if they cannot get enough air. Often they are afraid and anxious or seem confused. They may say that they feel dizzy or that their fingers and toes feel numb and tingly.

Hyperventilation often results from fear or anxiety and is most likely to occur in people who are tense and nervous. However, it can also be caused by head injuries; severe bleeding; or illnesses such as high fever, heart failure, lung disease and diabetic emergencies. Asthma and exercise also can trigger hyperventilation.

Allergic Reactions

Allergic reactions also can cause breathing problems. At first the reaction may appear to be just a rash and a feeling of tightness in the chest and throat, but this condition can become life threatening. The person's face, neck and tongue may swell, closing the airway.

A severe allergic reaction can cause a condition called *anaphylactic shock,* also known as *anaphylaxis.* During anaphylaxis, air passages may swell and restrict a person's breathing. Anaphylaxis can be brought on by insect stings, food, other allergens and certain medications. Signals of anaphylaxis include rashes; tightness in the chest and throat; and swelling of the face, neck and tongue. The person may also feel dizzy or confused. If not recognized early and cared for quickly, anaphylactic shock can become a life-threatening emergency.

Some people know that they are allergic to certain substances or to bee stings. They may have learned to avoid these things and may carry medication to reverse the allergic reaction. People who have severe allergic reactions may wear a medical alert tag.

For more information on allergic reactions and treatment for anaphylaxis, see Chapter 14.

Caring for Breathing Emergencies.

If a person's breathing is too fast, slow, noisy or painful, call 9-1-1 or the local emergency number immediately. Otherwise, if a person is having trouble breathing, help him or her rest in a comfortable position. Usually, sitting is more comfortable than lying down because breathing is easier in that position (Fig. 4-4). If the person is conscious, check for other conditions.

Remember that a person having breathing problems may find it hard to talk. If the person cannot talk, ask him or her to nod or shake his or her head to answer yes-or-no questions. Try to reassure the person and reduce anxiety. This may make his or her breathing easier. If there are bystanders and the person with trouble breathing is having trouble answering your questions, ask them what they know about the person's condition.

If the person is hyperventilating and you are sure it is caused by emo-

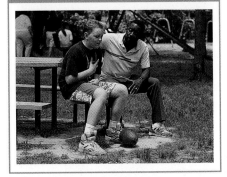

FIGURE 4-4 A person who is having trouble breathing may breathe more easily in a sitting position.

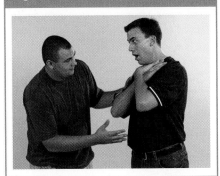

FIGURE 4-5 Clutching the throat with one or both hands is universally recognized as a signal for choking.

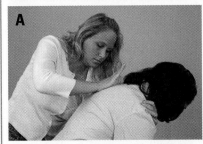

FIGURE 4-6, A-B If a conscious adult has a completely blocked airway, give back blows and abdominal thrusts.

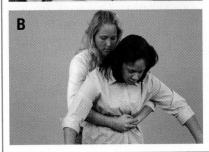

FIGURE 4-7, A-B If a conscious child has a completely blocked airway, give back blows and abdominal thrusts.

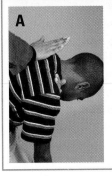
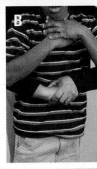

tion, such as excitement or fear, tell the person to relax and breathe slowly. A person who is hyperventilating from emotion may resume normal breathing if he or she is reassured and calmed down. If the person's breathing still does not slow down, the person could have a serious problem.

When breathing is too fast, slow, noisy or painful, call 9-1-1 or your local emergency number immediately.

Choking

Choking is a common breathing emergency. If a conscious person is choking, his or her airway has been blocked by a foreign object such as piece of food or a small toy, by swelling in the mouth or throat, or by fluids such as vomit or blood. The airway may be partially or completely blocked. With a partially blocked airway, the person usually can breathe with difficulty. A person whose airway is completely blocked cannot breathe at all.

A person with a partially blocked airway may be able to get enough air in and out of the lungs to cough or to make wheezing sounds. The person may also get enough air to speak. If the choking person is coughing force-

fully, let him or her try to cough up the object. A person who is getting enough air to cough or speak is getting enough air to breathe. Stay with the person and encourage him or her to continue coughing. However, if the person continues to cough without coughing up the object, have someone call 9-1-1 or the local emergency number.

Care for a Choking Emergency.
A partially blocked airway can very quickly become completely blocked. A person whose airway is completely blocked cannot cough, speak or breathe (Fig. 4-5). Sometimes the person may cough weakly or make high-pitched noises. This tells you the person is not getting enough air to stay alive. Act at once! If a bystander is available, have him or her call 9-1-1 or the local emergency number while you begin to give care.

Conscious Choking Adult or Child.
A conscious adult (Fig. 4-6, A-B) or child (Fig. 4-7, A-B) who has a completely blocked airway needs immediate care. A combination of 5 back blows followed by 5 abdominal thrusts provides an effective way to clear the airway obstruction.

To give back blows, position yourself slightly behind the person. Provide support by placing one arm diagonally across the chest and lean the person forward. Firmly strike the person between the shoulder blades with the heel of your other hand.

To give abdominal thrusts to a conscious choking adult or child—

- Stand or kneel behind the person and wrap your arms around his or her waist.
- Make a fist with one hand and place the thumb side against the middle of the person's abdomen, just above the navel and well below the lower tip of the breastbone.
- Grab your fist with your other hand and give quick, upward thrusts into the abdomen. Each back blow and abdominal thrust should be a separate and distinct attempt to dislodge the obstruction.
- Continue back blows and abdominal thrusts until the object is dislodged and the person can breathe or cough forcefully, or becomes unconscious.

Special Situations. If a conscious choking person is too big for you to reach around and give effective abdominal thrusts, such as a large or obviously pregnant person or someone known to be pregnant give chest thrusts instead (Fig. 4-8). Chest thrusts for a conscious adult are like abdominal thrusts, except for the placement of your hands. For chest thrusts, place your fist against the center of the person's breastbone. Then grab your fist with your other hand and give quick thrusts into the chest.

If you are alone and choking, lean over and press your abdomen against any firm object such as the back of a chair, a railing or the kitchen sink (Fig. 4-9). Do not lean over anything with a sharp edge or corner that might hurt you, and be careful when leaning on a rail that is elevated. Alternatively, give yourself abdominal thrusts, using your hands, just as if you were administering the abdominal thrusts to another person (Fig. 4-10).

For a choking victim in a wheelchair, give abdominal thrusts (Fig. 4-11).

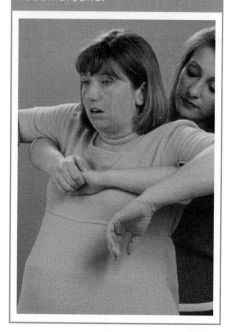

FIGURE 4-8 Give chest thrusts to a choking person who is pregnant or too big for you to reach around.

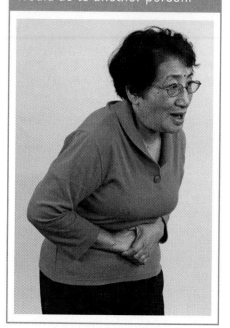

FIGURE 4-10 You can give yourself abdominal thrusts by using your hands, just as you would do to another person.

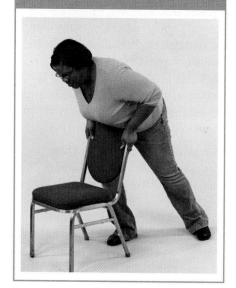

FIGURE 4-9 If you are alone and choking, lean over and press your abdomen against any firm object such as the back of a chair.

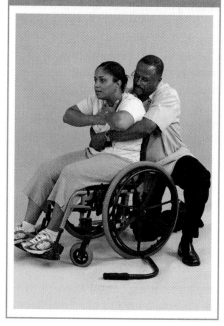

FIGURE 4-11 Give a choking victim in a wheelchair abdominal thrusts.

Conscious Choking Infant. An infant can easily swallow small objects, such as pebbles, coins, beads and parts of toys, which can then block the airway. Infants also often choke because their eating skills develop slowly. Therefore, they can easily choke on foods such as nuts, hot dogs, grapes and popcorn, which are often the perfect size to block their smaller airways.

If you determine that a conscious infant cannot cough, cry or breathe, you will need to give 5 back blows followed by 5 chest thrusts. To give back blows, follow these steps:

- Position the infant face-up on your forearm (Fig. 4-12, A).
- Place your other hand on top of the infant, using your thumb and fingers to hold the infant's jaw while sandwiching the infant between your forearms.
- Turn the infant over so that he or she is face-down on your forearm.
- Lower your arm onto your thigh so that the infant's head is lower than his or her chest. Then give 5 firm back blows with the heel of your hand between the infant's shoulder blades (Fig. 4-12, B). Each blow should be a separate and distinct attempt to dislodge the object.
- Maintain support of the infant's head and neck by firmly holding the jaw between your thumb and forefinger.

To give chest thrusts—

- Place the infant in a face-up position (Fig. 4-13, A).
- Place your free hand and forearm along the infant's head and back so that the infant is sandwiched between your two hands and forearms.
- Continue to support the infant's head between your thumb and finger from the front while you cradle the back of the head with your other hand.
- Turn the infant onto his or her back.

FIGURE 4-12, A-B A, To give back blows, position the infant face-up on your forearm. B, Then sandwich the infant between your forearms and support the head and neck by holding the jaw between your thumb and forefinger. Turn the infant over so that he or she is face-down on your forearm. Give 5 firm back blows with the heel of your hand while supporting the arm that is holding the infant on your thigh.

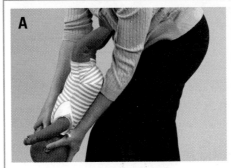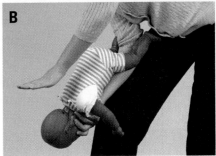

FIGURE 4-13, A-B A, To give chest thrusts, sandwich the infant between your forearms. Continue to support the infant's head. B, Turn the infant onto his or her back and support your arm on your thigh. The infant's head should be lower than its chest. Give 5 chest thrusts.

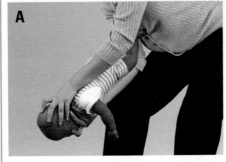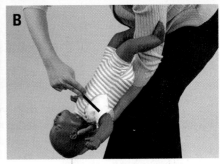

- Lower your arm that is supporting the infant's back onto your opposite thigh. The infant's head should be lower than his or her chest, which will assist in dislodging the object.
- Locate the correct place to give chest thrusts by imagining a line running across the infant's chest between the nipples.
- Place the pads of two or three fingers in the center of the infant's chest.

- Use the pads of these fingers to compress the breastbone. Compress the breastbone ½ to 1 inch and then let the breastbone return to its normal position. Keep your fingers in contact with the infant's breastbone.
- Using this method, give a total of 5 chest thrusts (Fig. 4-13, B).

Continue giving back blows and chest thrusts until the object is forced out, the infant begins to breathe on his or her own or the infant becomes unconscious.

PREVENTING CHOKING

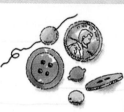

Don't leave small objects, such as buttons, coins and beads, within an infant's reach.

Have children sit in a high chair or at a table while they eat.

Do not let children eat too fast.

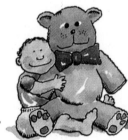

Give infants soft food that they do not need to chew.

Make sure that toys are too large to be swallowed.

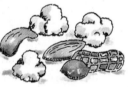

Do not give infants and young children foods like nuts, grapes, popcorn and raw vegetables.

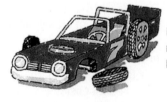

Make sure that toys have no small parts that could be pulled off.

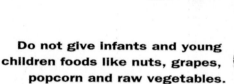

Cut foods a child can choke on easily, such as hot dogs, into small pieces.

Supervise children while they eat.

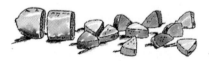

You can give back blows and chest thrusts effectively whether you stand or sit, as long as the infant is supported on your thigh. If the infant is large or your hands are too small to adequately support it, you may prefer to sit.

Rescue Breathing for Children.
When a child stops breathing, you have to breathe for that person. This is called rescue breathing. To give rescue breathing—

- Tilt the child's head back and lift the chin to move the tongue away from the back of the throat (Fig. 4-14). This opens the airway.
- Place your ear next to the person's mouth. Check for breathing by looking at the chest and listening and feeling for breathing, for no more than 10 seconds. If you cannot see, hear or feel any signs of breathing, begin breathing for the person.
- Pinch the nose shut and, after taking a breath, make a complete seal around the person's mouth with your mouth.

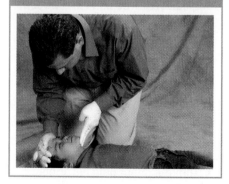

FIGURE 4-14 Tilt the child's head back and lift the chin to move the tongue away from the back of the throat.

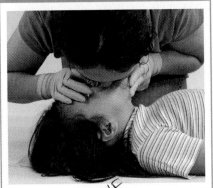

FIGURE 4-15 Breathe into the child until you see the chest clearly rise.

[handwritten note: BREATHE 1 - 1 THSD IN 2 THSD PAUSE BREATHE]

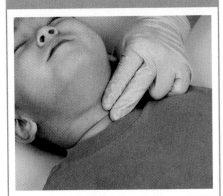

FIGURE 4-16 Check for a pulse after giving the 2 initial rescue breaths.

- Breathe into the child until you see the chest clearly rise (Fig. 4-15). Give 2 rescue breaths, each lasting about 1 second. Pause between rescue breaths to let the air flow out. Watch the child's chest clearly rise and fall each time you give a rescue breath.
- Check for a pulse after giving the 2 initial rescue breaths for no more than 10 seconds (Fig. 4-16).
- If there are signs of life but the child is still not breathing, give 1 rescue breath about every 3 seconds. A good way to time the rescue breaths is to count out loud, "one one thousand," take a breath on "two one thousand" and breathe into the child on "three one thousand."

After about 2 minutes, recheck for signs of life and pulse for no more than 10 seconds to make sure the heart is still beating. If there are signs of life but no breathing, continue rescue breathing. Continue rescue breathing until one of the following happens:
  - The scene becomes unsafe.

- The person begins to breathe on his or her own.
- You are too exhausted to continue.
- Another trained responder takes over for you.

If, at any time during your care, you do not see the child's chest clearly rise as you give rescue breaths, you might not have tilted the head far enough back. Reposition the child's airway by tilting the head farther back and repeat the breath. If your breaths still do not go in, the airway is probably blocked. You will learn how to clear a blocked airway of an unconcious person in Chapter 5.

Rescue Breathing for Infants. When an infant stops breathing, his or her body can function for only a few minutes without oxygen before body systems begin to fail. Like a child, an infant who is not breathing but shows another sign of life needs rescue breathing immediately.

To determine if you need to give rescue breaths, check the infant's breathing by tilting the head back with one hand and lifting the chin with the

FIGURE 4-17 Check the infant's breathing by tilting the head back with one hand and lifting the chin with two fingers on the chin.

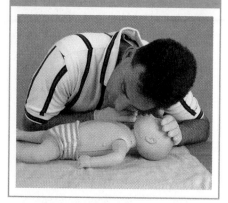

FIGURE 4-18 Give 2 rescue breaths.

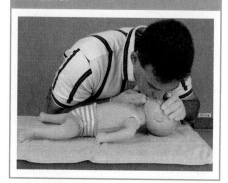

FIGURE 4-19 Check for a pulse for no more than 10 seconds.

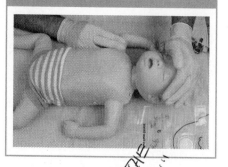

other hand (Fig. 4-17). Look, listen and feel for breathing for no more than 10 seconds. You do not need to tilt an infant's head back very far to open the airway.

If the infant is not breathing, you will have to give rescue breaths. Follow these steps:

- Take a breath, making a complete seal with your mouth over the infant's mouth and nose. Because an infant's mouth and nose are so small, it is easier to cover them both with your mouth than it is to pinch the nose.
- Give 2 rescue breaths (Fig. 4-18). Breathe into the infant only until you see the chest clearly rise. Each breath should last 1 second.
- Pause between rescue breaths to let the air flow back out. Watch the chest clearly rise each time you breathe in to be sure that your rescue breaths are actually going in.
- Check for a pulse for no more than 10 seconds (Fig. 4-19). In an infant, check for a pulse by pressing your first two fingers against the bone on the inside of the infant's upper arm between the elbow and the shoulder.
- If the infant is not breathing but has a pulse, continue rescue breathing. Give 1 rescue breath about every 3 seconds. A good way to time the breaths is to count out loud, "one one thousand," take a breath yourself on "two one thousand," and breathe into the infant on "three one thousand." Remember to breathe gently. Breathing too hard or too fast can force air into the infant's stomach.

If the infant has a pulse but is not breathing, continue rescue breathing. After 2 minutes of rescue breathing

(about 40 breaths), recheck the infant for breathing and other signs of life. Check for signs of life for no more than 10 seconds. If the infant still shows signs of life but is not breathing, continue rescue breathing until—

- The scene becomes unsafe.
- The infant begins to breathe on his or her own.
- You are too exhausted to continue.
- Another trained responder takes over for you.

If at any time during your care you do not see the infant's chest clearly rise as you give rescue breaths, you might not have positioned the head properly. Reposition the infant's airway by retilting the head and repeat the breaths. If your breaths still do not go in, the airway is probably blocked. You will learn how to clear a blocked airway in Chapter 5.

Breathing Barriers. You might not feel comfortable with the thought of giving rescue breathing, especially to someone you do not know. Disease transmission is an understandable worry, even though the chance of getting a disease from giving rescue breaths is extremely small.

CPR breathing barriers, such as face shields and resuscitation masks, create a barrier between your mouth and nose and the ill or injured person's (Fig. 4-20, A-B). This barrier can help protect you from contact with blood and other body fluids, such as saliva, as you give rescue breaths. These devices also protect you from breathing the air that the person exhales. Some devices are small enough to fit in your pocket or in the glove compartment of your car. You can also keep one in your first aid kit. If a face shield is used, switch to a resuscitation mask if available or when one becomes available. How-

FIGURE 4-20, A-B CPR breathing barriers, such as A, face shields and B, resuscitation masks, create a barrier between your mouth and nose and the ill or injured person's.

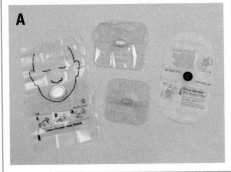

A

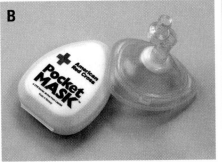

B

FIGURE 4-21 If you are unable to make a tight enough seal over the person's mouth, you can breathe into the nose.

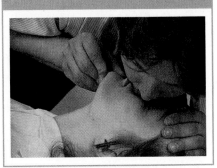

ever, you should *never delay* rescue breathing while searching for a breathing barrier or learning how to use one.

Special Situations

Air in the Stomach. When you are giving rescue breaths, be careful to avoid forcing air into the person's stomach instead of the lungs. This may happen if you breathe too long, breathe too hard or do not open the airway far enough.

To avoid forcing air into the person's stomach, keep the person's head tilted back. Take a normal breath, then breathe into the person, just enough to make the chest clearly rise. Each rescue breath should last about 1 second for an adult, child or infant. Pause between breaths long enough for the air in the person to come out and for you to take another breath.

Air in the stomach can make the person vomit and cause complications. When an unconscious person vomits, the contents of the stomach can get into the lungs and block breathing. Air

in the stomach also makes it harder for the diaphragm, the large muscle that controls breathing, to move. This makes it harder for the lungs to fill with air.

Vomiting. Even when you are giving rescue breaths properly, the person may vomit. If this happens, roll the person onto one side and wipe the mouth clean. If possible, use a protective barrier, such as disposable gloves, gauze or even a handkerchief, when cleaning out the mouth. Then roll the person on his or her back again and continue with rescue breathing if necessary.

Mouth-to-Nose and Stoma Breathing. If you are unable to make a tight enough seal over the person's mouth, you can breathe into the nose (Fig. 4-21). With the head tilted back, close the mouth by pushing on the chin. Seal your mouth around the person's nose and breathe into the nose. If possible, open the person's mouth between rescue breaths to let the air out.

On rare occasions, you may see an opening in a person's neck as you tilt the head back to check for breathing. This person may have had an operation to remove part of the windpipe. If so, the person breathes through this opening, which is called a *stoma,* instead of through the mouth or nose (Fig. 4-22). This person will probably have some form of medical identification, such as a bracelet, necklace or anklet, identifying this condition. Look, listen and feel for breathing with your ear over the stoma (Fig. 4-23, A). To give rescue breathing to this person, breathe into the stoma at the same rate you would breathe into the mouth (Fig. 4-23, B).

Submersion Victims. You should give 2 minutes of care before calling 9-1-1 *(Care First)* for an unconscious person who has been submerged. Get help from a trained responder to get the person out of the water as quickly and safely as possible. If the person is not breathing, you will have to breathe for him or her.

MAKE YOUR HOME SAFE FOR KIDS

Storage Areas

- Are pesticides, detergents and other household chemicals kept out of children's reach?
- Are tools kept out of children's reach?

General Safety Precautions Inside the Home

- Are stairways kept clear and uncluttered?
- Are stairs and hallways well lit?
- Are safety gates installed at tops and bottoms of stairways?
- Are guards installed around fireplaces, radiators, hot pipes and wood-burning stoves?
- Are sharp edges of furniture cushioned with corner guards or other material?
- Are curtain cords and shade pulls kept out of children's reach?
- Are fire extinguishers installed where they are most likely to be needed?
- Are smoke alarms installed and in working order? Are batteries changed at least every 6 months?
- Do you have an emergency plan to use in case of fire? Does your family practice this plan?
- Is the water set at a safe temperature? (A setting of 120° F or less prevents scalding from tap water in sinks and in tubs. Let the water run for 3 minutes before testing it.)
- If you have a gun, is it stored so that your child, and other unauthorized users, cannot use it?

- Are all purses, handbags, briefcases and similar items, including those belonging to visitors, kept out of children's reach?
- Are all poisonous plants kept out of children's reach?
- Is a list of emergency phone numbers posted near telephones?
- Is a list of instructions posted near telephones for use by children or babysitters?

Bathroom

- Are the toilet seat and lid kept down when the toilet is not in use?
- Are cabinets equipped with safety latches and kept closed?
- Are all medicines in child-resistant containers and stored in a locked medicine cabinet?
- Are shampoos and cosmetics stored out of children's reach?
- Are razors, razor blades and other sharp objects kept out of children's reach?
- Are hair dryers and other appliances stored away from the sink, tub or toilet?
- Does the bottom of tub or shower have non-slip surfacing?
- Are children always watched by an adult while in the bathroom?

Kitchen

- Do you cook on back stove burners when possible and turn pot handles toward the back of the stove?
- Are hot dishes kept away from the edges of tables and counters?
- Are hot liquids and foods kept out of children's reach?
- Are knives and other sharp items kept out of children's reach?
- Is the highchair placed away from stove and other hot appliances?
- Are matches and lighters kept out of children's reach?
- Are all appliance cords kept out of children's reach?
- Are cabinets equipped with safety latches?
- Are cleaning products kept out of children's reach?
- Do you test the temperature of heated food before feeding children?

Child's Room

- Is the bed or crib placed away from radiators and other hot surfaces?
- Are crib slats no more than $2\frac{3}{8}$ inches apart?
- Does the mattress fit the sides of the crib snugly?
- Is paint or finish on furniture and toys nontoxic?

- Is children's clothing, especially sleepwear, flame resistant?
- Does the toy box have secure lid and safe-closing hinges?
- Are electric cords kept out of children's reach?
- Are toys in good repair?
- Are toys appropriate for children's ages?

Parents' Bedroom

- Are space heaters kept away from curtains and flammable materials?
- Are cosmetics, perfumes and breakable items stored out of children's reach?
- Are small objects, such as jewelry, buttons and safety pins, kept out of children's reach?

Outside the Home

- Is trash kept in tightly covered containers?
- Are walkways, stairs and railings in good repair?
- Are walkways and stairs free of toys, tools and other objects?
- Are sandboxes and wading pools covered when not in use?
- Are nearby swimming pools enclosed with a fence that children cannot easily climb over?
- Is the backyard pool separated from the home's entrance by a fence?
- Is playground equipment safe? Is it assembled according to the manufacturer's instructions?

CHILD SAFETY IQ

- ☐ Do you buckle your child into an approved automobile safety seat in the back seat even when making short trips?
- ☐ Do you teach your child safety by behaving safely in your own everyday activities?
- ☐ Do you supervise your child whenever he or she is around water and maintain fences and gates that act as barriers to water?
- ☐ Have you checked your home for potential fire hazards?
- ☐ Are smoke detectors installed and working? Have you installed a carbon monoxide alarm?
- ☐ Are all poisonous substances, such as cleaning supplies, medicines and plants, kept out of children's reach?
- ☐ Are foods and small items that can choke a child kept out of reach?
- ☐ Have you inspected your home, daycare center, school, babysitter's home or wherever your child spends time for potential safety and health hazards?
- ☐ Do you keep guns and ammunition stored separately and locked up?

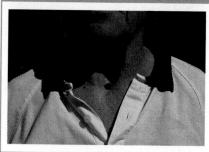

FIGURE 4-22 You may need to give rescue breaths to a person with a stoma, which is an opening in the front of the neck.

Hartman Films

Head, Neck and Back Injuries. Finally, be especially careful with a person who may have a head, neck or back injury. These kinds of injuries can result from a fall from a height greater than the person's, an automobile collision or a diving mishap. If you suspect such an injury, try not to move the person's head, neck and back. If a child is strapped into a car seat, do not remove him or her from it.

FIGURE 4-23, A-B A, To check for breathing, look, listen and feel for breaths with your ear over the stoma. B, To give rescue breaths, seal your mouth around the stoma and breathe into the person.

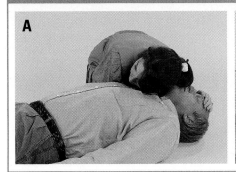

A

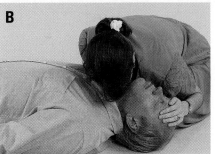

B

To care for a person who you suspect has a head, neck or back injury—

- Try to minimize movement of the head and neck when opening the airway.
- Tilt the head and lift the chin to open the airway.

Remember that the nonbreathing person's greatest need is for air. If a person's breathing stops or is restricted long enough, he or she will become unconscious and the heart will stop beating. Blood and oxygen will no longer circulate throughout the body. Other body systems will quickly fail.

Conscious Choking—Adult

STEP 1
CHECK scene, then **CHECK** person.

STEP 2
Have someone **CALL 9-1-1**.

STEP 3
Obtain consent.

STEP 4
Lean the person forward and give **5** back blows with the heel of your hand.

STEP 5
Give **5** quick, upward abdominal thrusts.

> *(**NOTE:** Give chest thrusts to a choking person who is pregnant or too big for you to reach around.)*

> *(**NOTE:** You can give yourself abdominal thrusts by using your hands, just as you would do to another person, or lean over and press your abdomen against any firm object such as the back of a chair.)*

STEP 6
Continue back blows and abdominal thrusts until—

- Object is forced out.
- Person can breathe or cough forcefully.
- Person becomes unconscious.

WHAT TO DO NEXT

IF PERSON BECOMES UNCONSCIOUS—
CALL 9-1-1, IF NOT ALREADY DONE, and give care for unconscious choking.

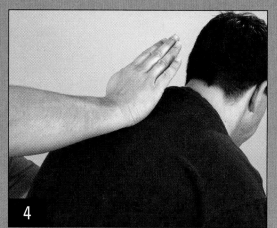

4

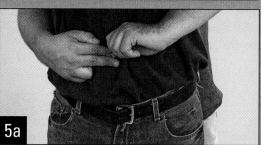

5a

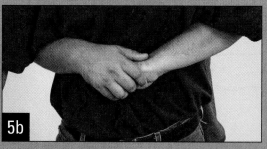

5b

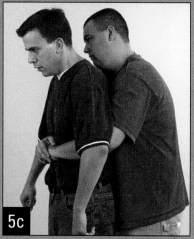

5c

Conscious Choking—Child

STEP 1
CHECK scene, then **CHECK** child.

STEP 2
Have someone **CALL 9-1-1**.

STEP 3
Obtain consent from parent or guardian, if present.

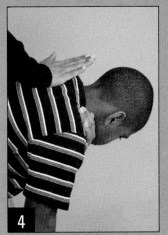

STEP 4
Lean the child forward and give **5** back blows with the heel of your hand.

STEP 5
Give **5** quick, upward abdominal thrusts.

(TIP: For a child, stand or kneel behind the child, depending on his or her size.)

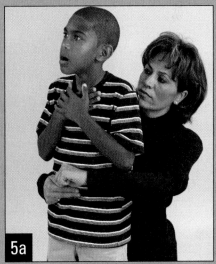

STEP 6
Continue back blows and abdominal thrusts until—
- Object is forced out.
- Child can breathe or cough forcefully.
- Child becomes unconscious.

WHAT TO DO NEXT
IF CHILD BECOMES UNCONSCIOUS—
CALL 9-1-1, IF NOT ALREADY DONE, and give care for unconscious choking.

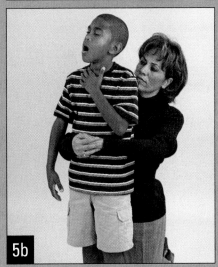

Conscious Choking—Infant

(CANNOT COUGH, CRY OR BREATHE)

STEP 1
CHECK scene, then CHECK infant.

STEP 2
Have someone CALL 9-1-1.

STEP 3
Obtain consent from parent or guardian, if present.

STEP 4
Give **5** back blows.

STEP 5
Give **5** chest thrusts.

(TIP: Hold head and neck securely when giving back blows and chest thrusts.)

STEP 6
Continue back blows and chest thrusts until—
- Object is forced out.
- Infant can breathe or cough forcefully.
- Infant becomes unconscious.

WHAT TO DO NEXT
IF INFANT BECOMES UNCONSCIOUS— CALL 9-1-1, IF NOT ALREADY DONE, and give care for unconscious choking.

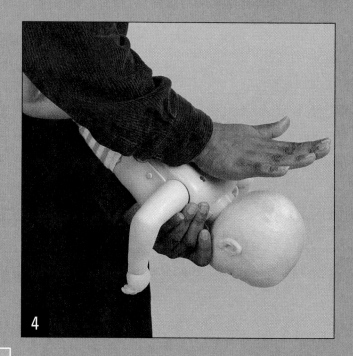

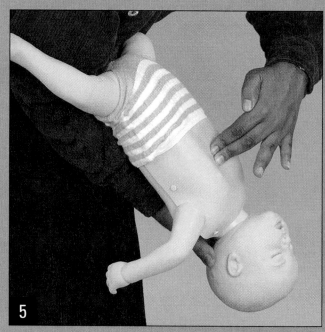

How to Give a Rescue Breath—Adult

After checking an ill or injured person

To give a rescue breath—

STEP 1

Tilt head and lift chin, then pinch the nose shut.

STEP 2

Take a breath and make a complete seal over the person's mouth.

STEP 3

Blow in to make chest clearly rise.

(TIP: Each rescue breath should last about 1 second.)

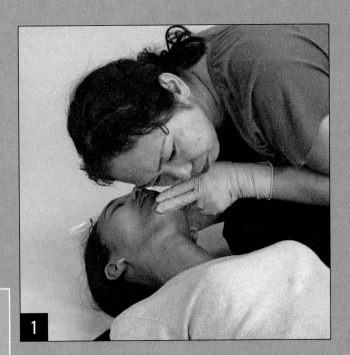

WHAT TO DO NEXT

IF BREATHS GO IN—Give CPR or use an AED (if AED is immediately available).

IF BREATHS DO NOT GO IN—Give care for unconscious choking.

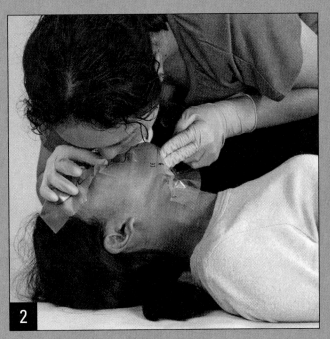

Rescue Breathing—Child

After checking an ill or injured child

STEP 1

Give **1** rescue breath about every **3** seconds.

- Pinch nose shut.
- Make seal over child's mouth.
- Blow in to make chest clearly rise.

*(**TIP:** Each rescue breath should last about 1 second.)*

*(**TIP:** Because children are smaller than adults, do not tilt the head back as far to open the airway.)*

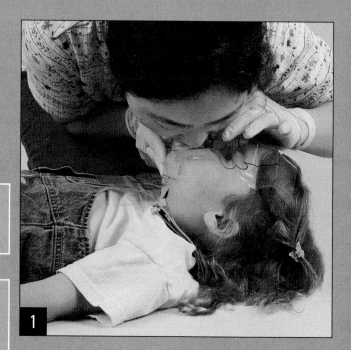

STEP 2

After about **2** minutes, recheck signs of life and pulse for no more than **10** seconds.

WHAT TO DO NEXT

IF PULSE, BUT NO BREATHING—Continue rescue breathing.

IF NO PULSE—Give CPR or use an AED (if AED is immediately available).

Rescue Breathing—Infant

After checking an ill or injured infant

STEP 1

Give **1** rescue breath about every **3** seconds.
Seal mouth over infant's mouth and nose.

> *(**TIP:** Each rescue breath should last about **1** second.)*

> *(**TIP:** Because infants are smaller than adults, do not tilt the head back as far to open the airway.)*

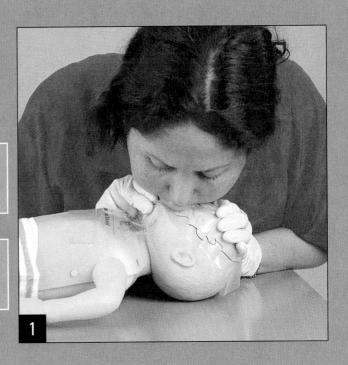

STEP 2

After about **2** minutes, recheck signs of life and pulse for no more than **10** seconds.

WHAT TO DO NEXT

IF PULSE, BUT NO BREATHING—Continue rescue breathing.

IF NO PULSE—Give CPR.

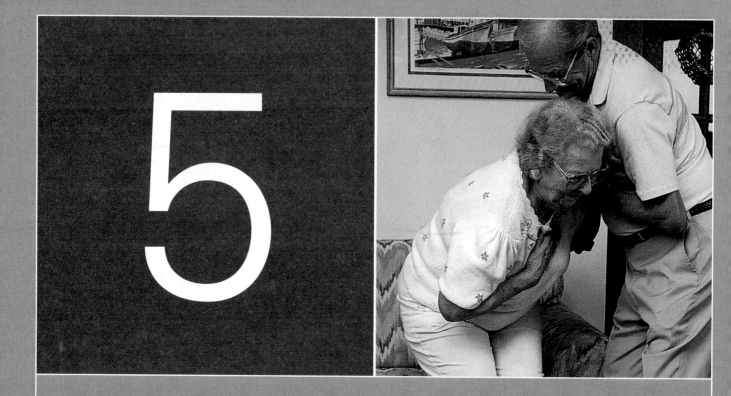

5

Any chest pain that is severe, lasts longer than 3 to 5 minutes or persists even during rest requires immediate medical care.

Chapter 5

Cardiac Emergencies

The heart is a fascinating organ. It beats more than 3 billion times in an average lifetime. The heart is about the size of a fist and lies between the lungs in the middle of the chest. It pumps blood throughout the body. The ribs, breastbone and spine protect it from injury. The heart is separated into right and left halves. Blood that contains little or no oxygen enters the right side of the heart and is pumped to the lungs. The blood picks up oxygen in the lungs when you breathe. The oxygen-rich blood then goes to the left side of the heart and is pumped to all parts of the body (Fig. 5-1).

Cardiovascular disease is an abnormal condition that affects the heart and blood vessels. An estimated 61 million Americans suffer from some form of cardiovascular disease. About 950,000 Americans die of cardiovascular disease each year. The main components of cardiovascular disease—*coronary heart disease*

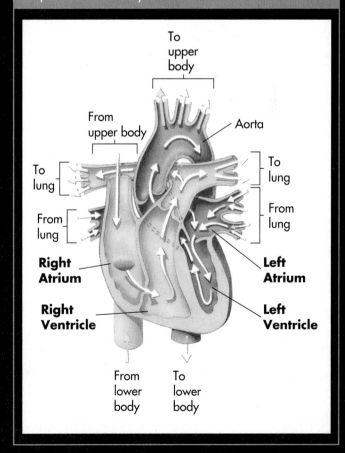

FIGURE 5-1 The heart is separated into right and left halves. Blood that contains little or no oxygen enters the right side of the heart and is pumped to the lungs. The blood picks up oxygen in the lungs when you breathe. The oxygen-rich blood then goes to the left side of the heart and is pumped to all parts of the body.

To upper body

From upper body

Aorta

To lung

To lung

From lung

From lung

Right Atrium

Left Atrium

Right Ventricle

Left Ventricle

From lower body

To lower body

and *stroke*—account for more than 40 percent of all deaths in the United States. Coronary heart disease is the most common type of cardiovascular disease.

The heart needs a constant supply of oxygen. Blood vessels called *arteries* supply the heart with oxygen-rich blood. Coronary heart disease occurs when fatty deposits containing cholesterol clog the arteries supplying the heart (Fig. 5-2). The arteries become less flexible and are not able to supply blood to the heart. If the heart does not get its blood, it will not work properly.

When the heart is working normally, it beats evenly and easily, with a steady rhythm. When damage to the heart causes it to stop working effectively, a person experiences a heart attack or other damage to the heart muscle. A heart attack can cause the heart to beat in an irregular way. This may prevent blood from circulating effectively. When the heart does not work properly, normal breathing can be disrupted or stopped. A heart attack can also cause the heart to stop beating entirely. This condition is called *cardiac arrest*. Although rare, children and teenagers can experience cardiac arrest.

WHEN THE HEART FAILS

The heart's electrical system sends out signals that tell the heart to pump blood. These signals travel through the upper chambers of the heart, called the *atria*, to the lower chambers, called the *ventricles*.

When the heart is normal and healthy, these electrical signals cause the ventricles to squeeze together, or contract. These contractions force blood out of the heart. The blood then circulates throughout the body. When the ventricles relax between contractions, blood flows back into the heart. The pause that you notice between heart beats when taking a person's pulse are the pauses between contractions.

If the heart is damaged by disease or injury, its electrical system can be disrupted. This can cause an abnormal heart rhythm that can stop the blood from circulating. The most common abnormal rhythm the heart goes into during sudden cardiac arrest is *ventricular fibrillation,* or V-fib. During V-fib, the heart's electrical signals stop making sense. This causes fibrillation, or quivering, of the ventricles. As a result, the ventricles do not contract, the heart cannot send enough blood through the body and there are no signs of life.

Another abnormal rhythm found during cardiac arrest is *ventricular tachycardia*, or V-tach. With V-tach, the electrical system tells the ventricles to contract too quickly. As a result, the heart cannot pump blood properly. As with V-fib, during V-tach the person will show no signs of life.

Defibrillation to the Rescue
In many cases, V-fib and V-tach rhythms can be corrected by an electric shock delivered by an automated external defibrillator (AED). This shock disrupts the abnormal electrical activity of V-fib and V-tach long enough to allow the heart to develop an effective rhythm on its own.

If V-fib or V-tach is not interrupted, the heart's electrical system, which may eventually stop working, may result in a condition called *asystole*. Asystole cannot be corrected by defibrillation and the person will die without further help. Therefore, it is important to start CPR immediately and continue until advanced medical help is available.

SIGNALS OF A HEART ATTACK

A heart attack has some common signals. You should be able to recognize the following signals so that you can give proper care:

- **Discomfort, pressure or pain.** The major signal is persistent discomfort, pressure or pain in the chest that does not go away. Unfortunately, it is not always easy to distinguish heart attack pain from the pain of indigestion, muscle spasms or other conditions. This often causes people to delay getting medical care. Brief, stabbing pain or pain that gets worse when you bend or breathe deeply is not usually caused by a heart problem.

The pain associated with a heart attack can range from discomfort to an unbearable crushing sensation in the chest. The person may describe it as pressure, squeezing, tightness, aching or heaviness in the chest. Many heart attacks start slowly, as mild pain or discomfort. Often the person feels discomfort or pain in the center of the chest (Fig. 5-3). It may spread to the shoulder, arm, neck, jaw or back. The discomfort or pain becomes constant. It is usually not relieved by resting, changing position or taking medicine.

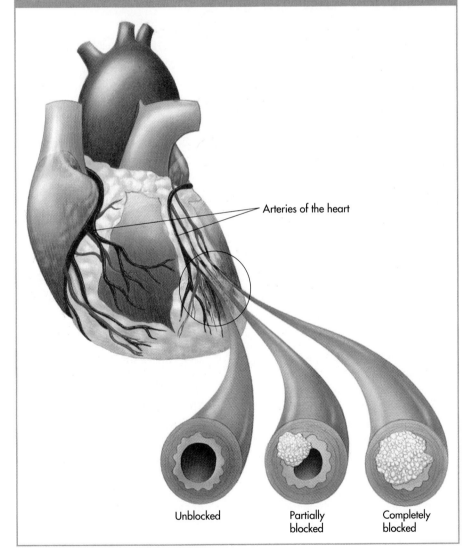

FIGURE 5-2 Buildup of fatty materials on the inner walls of the arteries reduces blood flow to the heart muscle and may cause a heart attack.

Arteries of the heart

Unblocked

Partially blocked

Completely blocked

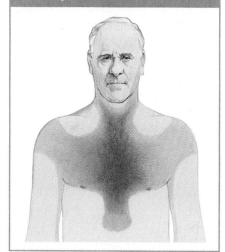

ASPIRIN CAN LESSEN HEART ATTACK DAMAGE

You may be able to help a conscious person who is showing early signals of a heart attack by offering him or her an appropriate dose of aspirin when the signals first begin. However, you should never delay calling 9-1-1 or the local emergency number to do this. Always call 9-1-1 or the local emergency number as soon as you recognize the signals, and then help the person to be comfortable before you give the aspirin.

Then, if the person is able to take medicine by mouth, ask if he or she—
- Is allergic to aspirin.
- Has a stomach ulcer or stomach disease.
- Is taking any blood thinners, such as Coumadin™ or Warfarin™.
- Has been told by a doctor not to take aspirin.

If the person answers no to all of these questions, you may offer him or her two chewable (162 mg) baby aspirins, or up to one 5-grain (325 mg) adult aspirin tablet with a small amount of water. Be sure that you only use aspirin and not Tylenol, acetaminophen, Motrin, Advil or ibuprofen, which are painkillers. Likewise, do not use coated aspirin products or products meant for multiple uses such as cold, fever and headache.

You may also offer these doses of aspirin if you have cared for the person and he or she has regained consciousness and is able to take the aspirin by mouth.

Any chest pain that is severe, lasts longer than 3 to 5 minutes, goes away and comes back or persists even during rest requires medical care at once. Even people who have had a heart attack may not recognize the signals, because each heart attack can have entirely different signals.
- **Pain that comes and goes.** Some people with coronary heart disease may have chest pain or pressure that comes and goes. This type of pain is called *angina pectoris*, a medical term for pain in the chest. It develops when the heart needs more oxygen than it gets because the arteries leading to it are too narrow. When a person with angina is exercising, excited or emotionally upset, the heart might not get enough oxygen. This lack of oxygen can cause chest discomfort or pain.

A person who knows he or she has angina may tell you so. People with angina usually have medicine to take to stop the pain. Stopping physical activity or easing the distress and taking the medicine usually ends the discomfort or pain of angina.
- **Trouble breathing.** Another signal of a heart attack is trouble breathing. The person may be breathing faster than normal because the body tries to get much-needed oxygen to the heart. The person's skin may be pale or ashen, especially around the face. The face also may be damp with sweat. Some people suffering from a heart attack sweat heavily or feel dizzy. These signals are caused by the stress put on the body when the heart does not work as it should.
- **Other signals.** Both men and women experience the most common signal for a heart attack, chest pain or discomfort. But women are somewhat more likely to experience some of the other warning signals, particularly

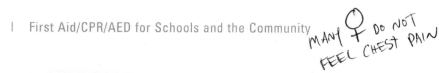
MANY ♀ DO NOT FEEL CHEST PAIN

shortness of breath, nausea or vomiting and back or jaw pain. Women also tend to delay telling others about their signals to avoid bothering or worrying them.
UNUSUAL FATIGUE

Prompt Action Is Key

It is important to recognize the signals of a heart attack and to act on those signals. Any heart attack might lead to cardiac arrest, but prompt action can often prevent the heart from stopping completely. A person suffering from a heart attack, and whose heart is still beating, has a far better chance of living than does a person whose heart has stopped. Most people who die of a heart attack die within 2 hours of the first signal. Many could have been saved if people on the scene or the person having the heart attack had been aware of the signals and acted promptly.

Early treatment with certain medications—including aspirin—can help minimize damage to the heart after a heart attack. To be most effective, these medications need to be given within 1 hour of the start of heart attack signals.

Many people who have heart attacks delay seeking care. Nearly half of all heart attack victims wait for 2 hours or more before going to the hospital. Often they do not realize they are having a heart attack. They may say the signals are just muscle soreness, indigestion or heartburn.

Remember, the key signal of a heart attack is chest discomfort or pain that does not go away. If the pain is severe, does not go away in 3 to 5 minutes or goes away and comes back, call 9-1-1 or the local emergency number at once. A person having a heart attack will probably deny that any signal is serious. Do not let this influence you. If you think the person might be having a heart attack, act quickly. Call 9-1-1 or the local emergency number immediately.

IN CASE OF A HEART ATTACK

If you suspect that someone might be having a heart attack, you should—

- Call 9-1-1 or the local emergency number at once.
- Have the person stop what he or she is doing and rest comfortably. This will ease the heart's need for oxygen. Many people experiencing a heart attack find it easier to breathe while sitting.
- Loosen any tight or uncomfortable clothing.
- Closely watch the person until EMS personnel arrive. Notice any changes in the person's appearance or behavior.
- Be prepared to give cardiopulmonary resuscitation (CPR) or use an AED if the person stops breathing and shows no other signs of life.

Talk to bystanders and the person to get more information. Ask the per-

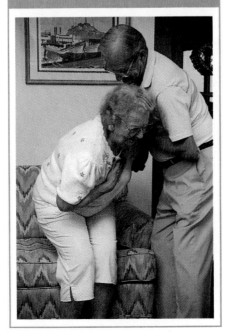

FIGURE 5-4 Comforting the person helps reduce anxiety and eases some of the discomfort.

son if he or she has a history of heart disease. Some people with heart disease take medication for chest pain. You can help by getting the medication for the person. Be calm and reassuring. Comforting the person helps reduce anxiety and eases some of the discomfort (Fig. 5-4). Do not try to drive the person to the hospital yourself. Her or she could quickly get worse on the way.

When the Heart Stops Beating

Cardiac arrest is the condition in which the heart stops beating or beats too ineffectively to circulate blood to the brain and other vital organs. Cardiac arrest is a life-threatening emergency because the body's vital organs are no longer receiving oxygen-rich blood. When cardiac arrest happens, breathing stops. Every year, more than 514,000 people die of cardiac arrest—more than 1400 Americans each day.

Cardiovascular disease is the most common cause of cardiac arrest. Other causes include drowning, choking, drugs, severe injury, brain damage, severe electric shock and chaotic electrical activity of the heart. Cardiac arrest can happen suddenly, without the signals usually seen in a heart attack.

The absence of signs of life is the main signal of cardiac arrest. No signs of life means no blood is going to the brain and other vital organs. Since blood carries oxygen, no oxygen is being supplied to the brain if a person is in cardiac arrest. Therefore, the brain will begin to die in a few minutes. A person in cardiac arrest will also be unconscious and not breathing.

Early CPR and Defibrillation

Even though a person is not breathing and shows no other signs of life, the cells of the brain and of other important organs continue to live for a short time—until all the oxygen in the blood is used. Such a person needs immediate *CPR* and *defibrillation*. CPR is a combination of chest compressions and rescue breathing. Defibrillation is a process of delivering an electrical shock that disrupts a heart's electrical activity long enough to allow the heart to spontaneously develop an effective rhythm on its own (Fig. 5-5).

As you read earlier, rescue breathing supplies oxygen. If a person shows signs of life, his or her heart is circulating this oxygen to the body through the blood. When the heart is not beating, chest compressions are needed to circulate the blood containing oxygen. Given together, rescue breaths and chest compressions take over for the heart and lungs. CPR increases the survival chances of a person in cardiac arrest by keeping

the brain and other vital organs supplied with oxygen until the person can receive defibrillation and advanced medical care. Without *early* CPR and *early* defibrillation, the chances of survival are greatly reduced.

Cardiac Chain of Survival ─VIDEO

CPR at best provides about one-third the normal blood flow to the brain. CPR alone is not enough to help someone survive cardiac arrest. Advanced medical care is needed as soon as possible. A person in cardiac arrest will have the greatest chance of survival from cardiac arrest if the following 4-step sequence called the "Cardiac Chain of Survival" occurs—

1. **Early recognition and early access.** The sooner someone calls 9-1-1 or the local emergency number, the sooner early advanced medical care arrives. This is why it is so important to call 9-1-1 or the local emergency number immediately.

2. **Early CPR.** Early CPR helps circulate blood that contains oxygen to the vital organs until an AED is ready to use or emergency medical personnel arrive.

3. **Early defibrillation.** Most victims of sudden cardiac arrest need an electric shock called *defibrillation*. Each minute that defibrillation is delayed reduces the chance of survival by about 10 percent.

4. **Early advanced medical care.** Trained medical personnel such as emergency medical technicians (EMTs) and paramedics provide further care and transport to hospital facilities.

In the Cardiac Chain of Survival, each link of the chain depends on and is connected to the other links. It is very important to recognize and start CPR promptly and continue it until an AED is available or EMS personnel arrive and take over. Any delay in calling 9-1-1 or the local emergency

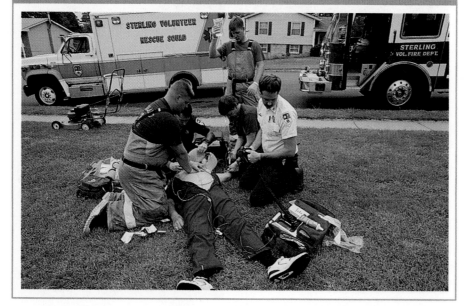

FIGURE 5-5 Defibrillation may help the heart to reestablish an effective heart rhythm.

PREVENTING CORONARY HEART DISEASE

Recognizing a heart attack and getting the necessary care at once may prevent a person from going into cardiac arrest. However, preventing a heart attack in the first place is even more effective. There is no substitute for prevention. Heart attacks are usually the result of disease of the heart and blood vessels. Coronary heart disease is the leading cause of death for adults in the United States. It accounts for nearly 500,000 deaths each year.

Coronary heart disease develops slowly. Deposits of cholesterol, a fatty substance made by the body and present in certain foods, build up on the inner walls of the arteries. The arteries gradually narrow. As the arteries that carry blood to the heart get narrower, less oxygen-rich blood flows to the heart. This reduced oxygen supply to the heart can eventually cause a heart attack.

Although a heart attack may seem to strike suddenly, many people live lives that are gradually putting their hearts in danger from coronary heart disease. Because coronary heart disease develops slowly, people may not be aware of it for many years. Fortunately, it is possible to slow the progress of coronary heart disease by making lifestyle changes.

Behavior that can harm the heart and blood vessels may begin in early childhood. We may develop a taste for "junk food," which is high in cholesterol and saturated fats but has little real nutritional value. Coronary heart disease can begin in the teens, especially if those are the years when people begin to smoke. Cigarette smoking greatly contributes to coronary heart disease and to other diseases.

Many things increase a person's chances of developing coronary heart disease. These are called *risk factors*. Some of them you cannot change. For instance, although more women than men die each year from coronary heart disease in the United States, heart disease generally affects men at younger ages than it does women.

Besides gender, ethnicity also plays an important role in determining the risk for heart disease. African Americans and Native Americans in the United States have higher rates of heart disease than do other populations. A history of heart disease in your family also increases your risk.

Altering Risk Factors

Many risk factors can be altered, however. Cigarette smoking, uncontrolled high blood cholesterol or high blood pressure, being overweight and not exercising regularly all increase the risk of heart disease. When you combine one risk factor, like smoking, with others, such as high blood pressure and not enough exercise, your risk of heart attack is much greater.

By taking steps to control your risk factors, you can improve your chances for living a long and healthy life. Remember, it is never too late.

It is important to know how to perform CPR and use an AED. However, the best way to deal with cardiac arrest is to prevent it. If you go into cardiac arrest, your chances of surviving are poor. Begin to reduce your risk of heart disease today.

number, starting CPR and using an AED makes it less likely the person will survive. Remember, you, the lay responder, are the first link in the Cardiac Chain of Survival.

CPR for Adults

To determine if an unconscious adult needs CPR, follow the emergency action steps (**CHECK—CALL—CARE**) that you learned in Chapter 2.

1. **CHECK** the scene and the ill or injured person.
2. **CALL** 9-1-1 or the local emergency number.
3. **CHECK** for breathing for no more than 10 seconds. If the person is not breathing, give 2 rescue breaths.
4. If there are no signs of life (movement or breathing), give **CARE** by giving CPR.

For chest compressions to be the most effective, the person should be on his or her back on a firm, flat surface. The person's head should be on the same level as the heart or lower. If the person is on a soft surface like a sofa or bed, move him or her to a firm surface before you begin.

To perform CPR on an adult—

- Locate the correct hand position by placing the heel of one hand on the person's sternum (breastbone) at the center of his or her chest (Fig. 5-6). Place your other hand directly on top of the first hand and try to keep your fingers off the chest by interlacing them or holding them upward (Fig. 5-7). If you have arthritis, you can give compressions by grasping the wrist of the hand positioned on the chest with your other hand (Fig. 5-8). The person's clothing should not interfere with finding the proper hand position, but if it does, remove any clothing covering the person's chest. The correct hand position allows you to give the most effec-

FIGURE 5-6 Locate the correct hand position by placing the heel of one hand on the person's sternum (breastbone) in the center of the person's chest.

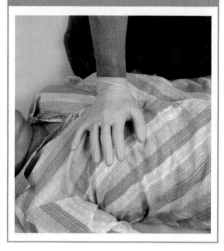

tive compressions without further injuring the person.

- Position your body correctly by kneeling beside the person, placing your hands in the correct posi-

FIGURE 5-8 If you have arthritis, you can give compressions by grasping the wrist of the hand positioned on the chest with your other hand.

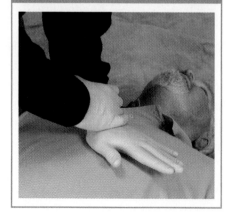

FIGURE 5-7 Place your other hand directly on top of the first hand. Try to keep your fingers off the chest by interlacing them or holding them upward.

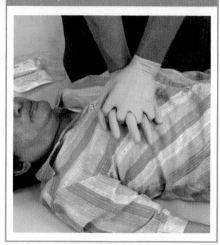

tion, straightening your arms and locking your elbows so that your shoulders are directly over your hands (Fig. 5-9). Your body position is important when providing chest

FIGURE 5-9 Position yourself so your shoulders are directly over your hands.

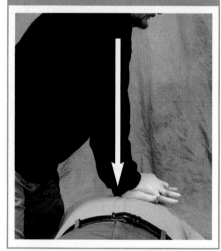

compressions. Compressing the person's chest straight down provides the best blood flow. The correct body position is also less tiring for you.

- Give compressions by pushing the sternum down from 1½ to 2 inches (Fig. 5-10). The downward and upward movement should be smooth, not jerky. Maintain a steady down-and-up rhythm, and do not pause between compressions. Spend half of the time pushing down and half of the time coming up. When you press down, the walls of the heart squeeze together, forcing the blood to empty out of the heart. When you come up, you should release all pressure on the chest. This allows the heart's chambers to fill with blood between compressions. Keep your hands in their correct position on the breastbone.

- Push straight down with the weight of your upper body, not with your arm muscles. This way, the weight of your upper body will create the force needed to compress the chest. Push straight down. Do not rock back and forth. Rocking results in less-effective compressions and wastes much-needed energy. If your arms and shoulders tire quickly, you are not using the correct body position.

- After each compression, release the pressure on the chest without removing your hands or changing hand position. Allow the chest to return to its normal position before starting the next compression.

- Give 30 compressions in about 18 seconds (or about 100 compressions per minute). 100 compressions per minute refers to the *speed of compressions,* not the *number of compressions* given in a minute. As you give compressions, count out loud, "One and two and three and four and five and six and…" up to 30. Push down as you say the number and come up as you say "and." This will help you keep a steady, even rhythm.

- Give 30 compressions, then open the airway using the head tilt/chin-lift technique and give 2 res-

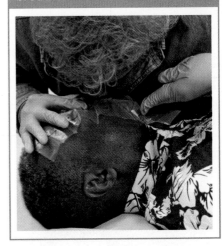

FIGURE 5-11 Give 2 rescue breaths.

cue breaths (Fig. 5-11). This cycle should take about 24 seconds.

- Continue cycles of CPR until an AED becomes available or EMS arrives and takes over (Fig. 5-12). If there are no signs of life, continue CPR, starting with 30 compressions. Continue CPR until an obvious sign of life is found or EMS personnel arrive and take over.

- If the person is breathing, keep his or her airway open and monitor breathing and signs of life closely until EMS personnel arrive (Fig. 5-13).

Special Considerations

Two Responders Available
If two responders trained in CPR are at the scene, you should both identify yourselves as being trained. One should call 9-1-1 or the local emergency number for help, if this has not been done, while the other gives CPR. If the first responder is tired and needs help—

- The first responder should tell the second responder to take over.

- The second should immediately resume CPR, beginning with chest compressions (Fig. 5-14).

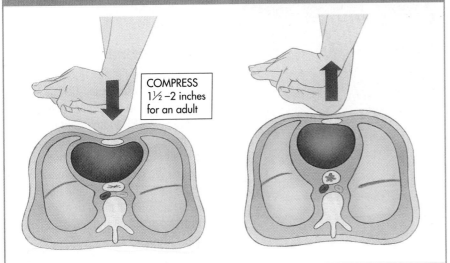

FIGURE 5-10 Push straight down with the weight of your body, then release, allowing the chest to return to the normal position.

COMPRESS
1½–2 inches
for an adult

FIGURE 5-12 Give CPR until an AED becomes available or EMS personnel arrive and take over.

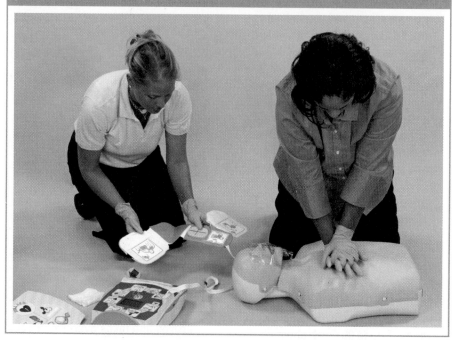

FIGURE 5-13 Monitor ABCs until help arrives.

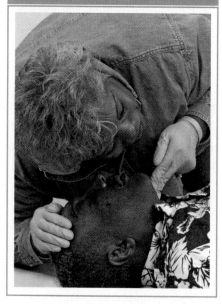

FIGURE 5-14 The second responder should take over CPR beginning with chest compressions.

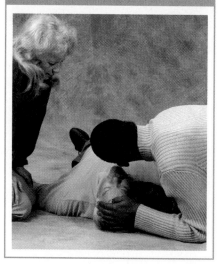

When to Stop CPR

Once you begin CPR, you should try not to interrupt the blood flow being created by your compressions. However, you can stop CPR if—

- The scene becomes unsafe.
- The person shows signs of life.
- An AED becomes available and is ready to use.
- Another trained responder arrives and takes over.
- You are too exhausted to continue.

CARDIAC EMERGENCIES IN CHILDREN AND INFANTS

Unlike adults, children do not often initially suffer a cardiac emergency. In general, a child or infant suffers a respiratory emergency and then a cardiac emergency develops. Motor vehicle crashes, drowning, smoke inhalation, poisoning, airway obstruction, firearm injuries and falls are all common causes of respiratory emergencies that can develop into a cardiac emergency. A cardiac emergency can also result from an acute respiratory condition, such as an asthma attack. If you recognize that an infant or child is in respiratory distress or respiratory arrest, give the care you learned in Chapter 4.

CPR for Children and Infants

As you would do for an adult, follow the emergency action steps (CHECK—CALL—CARE) to determine if you will need to give CPR to an infant or child. Remember that the CPR techniques you use will be slightly different because infants and children have smaller bodies and faster breathing and heart rates (Fig. 5-15). You will need to adjust your hand position and the depth of compressions.

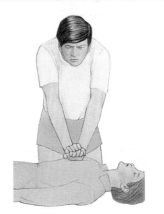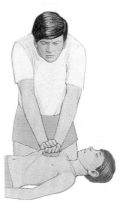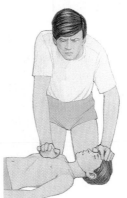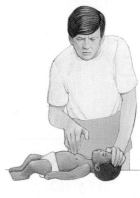

CPR SKILL COMPARISON CHART

Skill Components	Adult	Child	Infant
HAND POSITION:	Two hands in center of chest (on lower half of sternum)	One or two hands in center of chest (on lower half of sternum)	Two or three fingers on lower half of chest (one finger width below nipple line)
COMPRESS:	1½ to 2 inches	1 to 1½ inches	½ to 1 inch
BREATHE:	Until the chest rises (about 1 second per breath)	Until the chest rises (about 1 second per breath)	Until the chest rises (about 1 second per breath)
CYCLE:	30 compressions 2 breaths	30 compressions 2 breaths	30 compressions 2 breaths
RATE:	30 compressions in about 18 seconds (100 compressions per minute)	30 compressions in about 18 seconds (100 compressions per minute)	30 compressions in about 18 seconds (100 compressions per minute)

CPR for a Child. To find out if an unconscious child needs CPR, start by checking for life-threatening conditions. If you find that the child has no signs of life, including a pulse, place the child on a firm, flat surface and begin CPR by following these steps:

- Locate the proper hand position on the middle of the breastbone as you would for an adult (Fig. 5-16, A).
- Alternatively, you can use a one-handed technique by placing one hand on the child's chest and the other hand on the forehead to maintain an open airway (Fig. 5-16, B).
- Place your shoulder over your hand.

- Compress the chest smoothly to a depth of about 1½ inches using the heel of the dominant hand.
  - Lift up, allowing the chest to fully return to its normal position, but keep contact with the chest.
  - Repeat compressions, performing 30 compressions in about 18 seconds.
  - After giving 30 compressions, remove your compression hand(s) from the chest, open the airway and give 2 rescue breaths (Fig. 5-16, C). Each breath should last about 1 second. Use the head-tilt/chin-lift technique to ensure that the

child's airway is open.
  - After giving the breaths, place your hand(s) in the same position as before and continue compressions.

Keep repeating the cycles of 30 compressions and 2 rescue breaths. Continue CPR until an AED becomes available or EMS arrives and takes over.

If at any time the child starts breathing, keep the airway open, and monitor breathing and signs of life closely. If the child has a pulse but is not breathing, give rescue breathing and keep checking for signs of life and pulse about every 2 minutes.

FIGURE 5-16, A-C To give CPR to a child, A, Locate the proper hand position in the center of the child's chest by placing 2 hands on the center of the child's chest. B, Alternatively, place one hand on the child's chest and the other hand on the forehead to maintain an open airway. C, After giving 30 compressions, remove your compression hands from the chest, open the airway and give 2 rescue breaths.

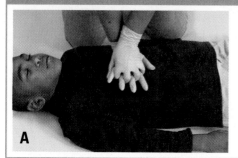
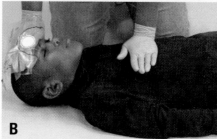
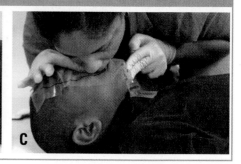

CPR for an Infant. To find out if an infant needs CPR, begin by checking for life-threatening conditions. Start by checking the infant for signs of life and a pulse. Position the infant face-up on a firm, flat surface. The infant's head must be on the same level as the heart or lower. Stand or kneel facing the infant from the side. Bare the infant's chest. Keep your hand on the infant's head to maintain an open airway. Use the fingers of your other hand to give compressions.

To find the correct location for compressions—

- Place the pads of two or three fingers below an imaginary line running across the chest between the nipples. Place the pads of these fingers on the middle of the chest (sternum) (Fig. 5-17, A). If you feel the notch at the end of the infant's sternum, move your fingers slightly toward the infant's head.
- Use the pads of these fingers to compress the chest. Compress the chest ½ to 1 inch. Push straight down (Fig. 5-17, B). Your compressions should be smooth, not jerky.
- Keep a steady rhythm. Do not pause between compressions except to give breaths. When your fingers are coming up, release pressure on the infant's chest

completely, but do not let your fingers lose contact with the chest. Compress at a rate of 100 compressions per minute.
- When you complete 30 compressions, give 2 rescue breaths, covering the infant's mouth and nose with your mouth (Fig. 5-17, C). Each breath should last about 1 second. Keep repeating cycles of 30 compressions and 2 breaths. Continue CPR until EMS personnel arrive and take over.

If you do find signs of life, then check breathing. If the infant is breathing, keep the airway open and monitor breathing and signs of life closely.

FIGURE 5-17, A-C To give CPR to an infant, A, place the pads of two or three fingers in the center of the infant's chest. Use the pads of two fingers to compress the chest. B, Compress the chest ½ to 1 inch deep. Push straight down. C, Give 2 rescue breaths, covering the infant's mouth and nose with your mouth.

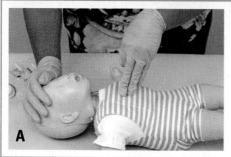
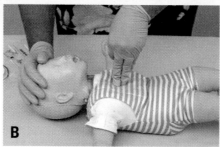
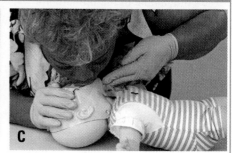

Recheck signs of life every few minutes. *Place an infant in a recovery position* as you would for an adult or child. If the infant has a pulse but is not breathing, give rescue breathing and check for signs of life and pulse about every 2 minutes.

Care for an Unconscious Choking Adult or Child

During your check for life-threatening conditions, you may discover that an unconscious person is not breathing and the 2 rescue breaths you give do not go in. In this case, reposition the person's airway by retilting the head and try 2 breaths again. You may not have tilted the person's head far enough back the first time. If the breaths still will not make the chest rise, assume that the person's airway is obstructed. To care for an unconscious adult or child with an airway obstruction, perform a modified CPR technique—

- Locate the correct hand position for chest compressions. Use the same techniques that you learned in CPR.
- Perform chest compressions. Compress an adult's chest to a depth of about 2 inches 30 times in about 18 seconds (Fig. 5-18, A). Compress a child's chest to a depth of about 1½ inches 30 times in about 18 seconds.
- Look for a foreign object (Fig. 5-18, B). Open the person's mouth. (Remove the CPR breathing barrier if you are using one.) If you see an object, remove it with your finger (Fig. 5-18, C).
- Give 2 rescue breaths (Fig. 5-18, D). If the breaths do not go in (chest does not rise), repeat cycles of chest compressions, foreign object check and 2 rescue breaths until—
  - The object is removed and the chest clearly rises with rescue breaths.

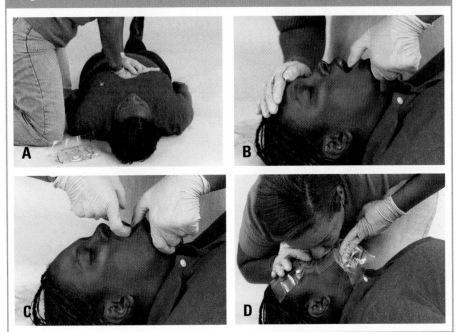

FIGURE 5-18, A-D For an unconscious choking adult, A, Compress the person's chest to a depth of about 2 inches. B, Look inside the person's mouth for an object. C, If you find one, remove it with your finger. D, Give 2 rescue breaths.

  - The person starts to breathe on his or her own.
  - EMS personnel or another trained responder arrive and take over.
  - You are too exhausted to continue.
  - The scene becomes unsafe.

If the breaths go in (the chest clearly rises), check for signs of life including a pulse for children, for no more than 10 seconds. Care for the conditions you find.

Care for an Unconscious Choking Infant

If you determine that an infant is unconscious, not breathing and you cannot get air into the lungs, reposition the airway by retilting the head and try 2 more rescue breaths. If you still cannot get air into the infant, assume that the airway is obstructed. To care for an unconscious infant with an airway obstruction—

- Locate the correct hand position for chest compressions. Use the same techniques that you learned in CPR.
- Give 30 chest compressions in about 18 seconds (Fig. 5-19, A). Each compression should be about ½ to 1 inch deep.
- Look for a foreign object (Fig. 5-19, B). If the object is seen, remove it with your little finger (Fig. 5-19, C).
- Give 2 rescue breaths (Fig. 5-19, D). If the breaths do not go in (chest clearly rises), repeat cycles of chest compressions, foreign object check and rescue breaths until—
  - The scene becomes unsafe.
  - The object is removed and the chest clearly rises with rescue breaths.

FIGURE 5-19, A-D For an unconscious choking infant, A, Give 30 chest compressions. B, Look for an object. C, If you find one, remove it with a smaller finger. D, Give 2 rescue breaths.

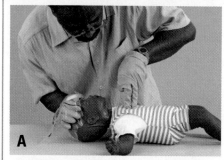
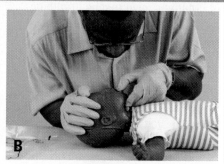
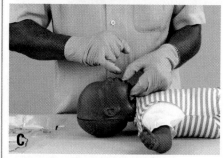
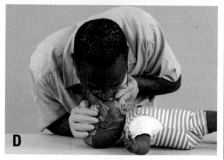

- ○ The infant starts to breathe on his or her own.
- ○ EMS personnel or another trained responder arrive and take over.
- ○ You are too exhausted to continue.

If the breaths go in (the chest clearly rises), check for signs of life, including a pulse, for no more than 10 seconds. Care for the conditions you find.

1ST CHECK CALL CARE

USING AN AED—ADULTS

As mentioned earlier, most people in sudden cardiac arrest need an electric shock called defibrillation. Each minute that defibrillation is delayed, the chances of survival are reduced by about 10 percent. Therefore, the sooner the shock is administered, the greater the chances are that the person will

survive. By learning how to use an AED, you can make a difference before EMS personnel arrive (Fig. 5-20).

An AED should be used as soon as it is available and safe to do so. However, as you learned in the Cardiac Chain of Survival, you should always call 9-1-1 or the local emergency number first. CPR in progress is stopped only when the AED is ready to analyze. Most AEDs can be operated by following these simple steps:

1. Turn on the AED (Fig. 5-21, A).
2. Wipe the person's bare chest dry. Apply the pads to the person's bare chest. Place one pad on the upper right chest and the other pad on the lower left side (Fig. 5-21, B).
3. Plug the connector into the AED, if necessary.
4. Let the AED analyze the heart rhythm (or push the button

Automated External Defibrilators

FIGURE 5-20 There are several types of AEDs.

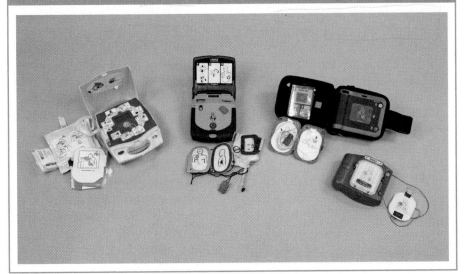

FIGURE 5-21, A-D To use an AED on an adult, A, Turn on the AED. B, Apply the pads to the person's bare chest. Place one pad on the upper right chest and the other pad on the lower left side. C, Let the AED analyze the heart rhythm. D, Deliver a shock by pushing the shock button if indicated and prompted by the AED.

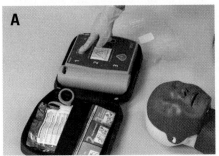
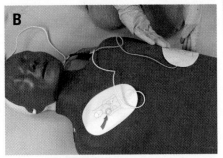
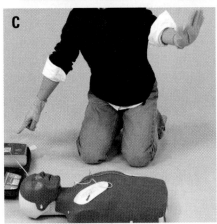
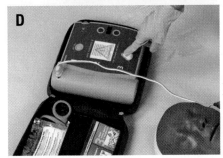

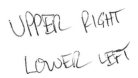

marked "analyze," if indicated and prompted by the AED) (Fig. 5-21, C).

○ Advise all responders and bystanders to "Stand clear."

○ Do not touch the person.

5. Deliver a shock by pushing the button if indicated and prompted by the AED (Fig. 5-21, D). Ensure that no one, including you, is touching the person and that there are no hazards present (such as puddles of water).

○ If the AED tells you "No shock advised," you may have to continue CPR.

In some cases, defibrillation is not required and the AED will not prompt you to deliver a shock. If no shock is indicated, leave the AED attached to the person and continue CPR for 5 cycles (or about 2 minutes). Continue care as needed.

USING AN AED—CHILDREN

Sudden cardiac arrest can happen to anyone, at any time and not just to adults. While the incidence is relatively low compared with adults, cardiac arrest resulting from ventricular fibrillation (V-fib) does happen to young children and infants and is no less dramatic. The emotional trauma and devastation of the loss of a child to a family and community cannot be measured.

Most cardiac arrests in children are not sudden. The most common causes of cardiac arrest in children are due to—

- Airway and breathing problems.
- Traumatic injuries or an accident (e.g., automobile, drowning, electrocution or poisoning).
- A hard blow to the chest. (e.g., *commotio cordis*).
- Congenital heart disease.

- Sudden Infant Death Syndrome (SIDS).

AEDs equipped with pediatric AED pads are capable of delivering lower levels of energy to a child between 1 and 8 years of age or weighing less than 55 pounds. Use the same general steps and precautions that you would when using an AED on an adult or a child in cardiac arrest.

1. Turn on the AED (Fig. 5-22, A).
2. Wipe the child's bare chest dry. *Make sure that you are using pediatric AED pads.* Apply the pads to the child's bare chest. Place one pad on the child's upper right chest and the other pad on the lower left side (Fig. 5-22, B). Make sure the pads are not touching. If the pads risk touching each other, place one pad on the child's chest and the other pad on the child's back (Fig. 5-22, C).
3. Plug the connector into the AED, if necessary.
4. Let the AED analyze the heart rhythm (or push the button marked "analyze," if indicated and prompted by the AED) (Fig. 5-22, D).
   - Advise all responders and bystanders to "Stand clear."
   - Do not touch the child.
5. Deliver a shock by pushing the button if indicated and prompted by the AED (Fig. 5-22, E). Ensure that no one, including you, is touching the child and that there are no hazards present (such as puddles of water).
   - If the AED tells you "No shock advised," you may have to continue CPR.

FIGURE 5-22, A-E To use an AED on a child. A, Turn on the AED. B, Place one pediatric pad on the upper right chest and the other pad on the lower left side. C, If the pads risk touching each other, place one on the child's chest and the other on the child's back. D, Let the AED analyze the heart rhythm. E, Deliver a shock by pushing the shock button if prompted by the AED.

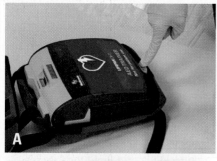
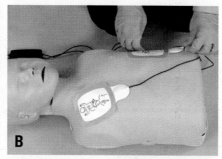
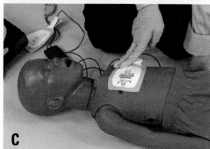
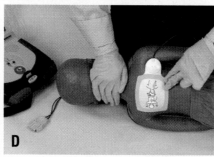
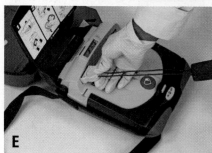

AED Precautions

When operating an AED, you should avoid certain actions and situations that could harm you, other responders, bystanders or the person in cardiac arrest. Always take the following precautions:

- Do not touch the person while the AED is analyzing. Touching or moving the person may affect the analysis.
- Do not touch the person while the device is defibrillating. You or others could be shocked.
- Prior to shocking a person with an AED, make sure that no one is touching or is in contact with the person or the resuscitation equipment.
- Do not use alcohol to wipe the person's chest dry. Alcohol is flammable.
- Do not defibrillate someone when around flammable materials

such as gasoline or free-flowing oxygen.

- Do not use an AED in a moving vehicle. Movement may affect the analysis.
- Do not use an AED on a person who is in contact with water. Move people away from puddles of water or swimming pools, or out of the rain before defibrillating.
- Do not use an AED and/or electrode pads designed for adults on a child under age 8 or less than 55 pounds unless pediatric pads specific to the device are not available. Local protocols may differ on this and should be followed.
- Do not use an AED on a person wearing a nitroglycerin patch or other patch on the chest. With a gloved hand, remove any patches from the chest before attaching the device.
- Do not use a cellular phone or radio within 6 feet of the AED. This may interrupt analysis.

Special AED Situations

Some situations require you to pay special attention when using an AED. Be familiar with these situations and know how to respond appropriately. Always use common sense when using an AED and follow the manufacturer's recommendations.

Wet Environments. If a person has been removed from water, dry the person's chest and attach the AED. The person should not be in a puddle of water, nor should the rescuer be kneeling in a puddle of water when operating an AED.

If it is raining, take steps to ensure that the person is as dry as possible and sheltered from the rain. Ensure that the person's chest is wiped dry. Minimize delaying defibril-

lation, though, when taking steps to provide for a dry environment. The electrical current of an AED is very directional between the electrode pads. AEDs are very safe, even in rain and snow, when all precautions and manufacturer's operating instructions are followed.

Implantable Devices. Some people whose hearts are weak and may beat too slow, skip beats or beat in a rhythm that is too fast may have had a pacemaker implanted. These small implantable devices are sometimes located in the area below the right collarbone. There may be a small lump that can be felt under the skin. Sometimes the pacemaker is placed somewhere else. Other individuals may have an implantable cardioverter-defibrillator (ICD), a miniature version of an AED, which acts to automatically recognize and restore abnormal heart rhythms. Sometimes, a person's heart beats irregularly, even if the person has a pacemaker or ICD.

If it is visible or you know that the person has an implanted device, do not place the defibrillation pads directly over the device (Fig. 5-23). This may interfere with the delivery of the shock. Adjust pad placement if necessary and continue to follow the established protocol. If you are not sure, use the AED if needed. It will not harm the person or responder.

Nitroglycerin Patches. People with a history of cardiac problems may have nitroglycerin patches on their chests. Since nitroglycerin can be absorbed by a responder, you should remove it with a gloved hand before defibrillation. Nicotine patches used to stop smoking look similar to nitroglycerin patches. In order not to waste time trying to identify patches, remove any patch you see on the person's chest.

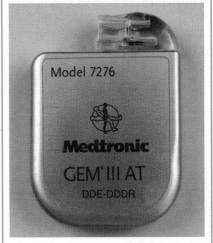

FIGURE 5-23 Look for an implantable cardioverter-defibrillator (ICD) before defibrillation.

Model 7276

Medtronic
GEM III AT
DDE-DDDR

Photo courtesy of Medtronic, Inc.

Hypothermia. Some people who have experienced hypothermia have been resuscitated successfully even after prolonged exposure. It will take longer to do your check, or assessment, of the person since you may have to check for signs of life and/or pulse for up to 30 to 45 seconds. If you do not feel a pulse, begin CPR until an AED becomes readily available. If the person is wet, dry his or her chest and attach the AED. If there is still no pulse, continue CPR. Follow local protocols as to whether additional shocks should be delivered. Continue CPR and protect the person from further heat loss. CPR or defibrillation should not be withheld to re-warm the person. Rescuers should take care not to shake a hypothermia victim unnecessarily as this could result in V-fib.

Trauma. If a person is in cardiac arrest resulting from traumatic injuries, an AED may still be used. Defibrillation should be administered according to local protocols.

AED Maintenance

For defibrillators to perform optimally, they must be maintained like any other machine. AEDs require minimal maintenance. These devices have various self-testing features. However, it is important that operators are familiar with any visual or audible warning prompts the AED may have to warn of malfunction or a low battery. It is important that you read the operator's manual thoroughly and check with the manufacturer to obtain all necessary information regarding maintenance.

In most instances, if the machine detects any malfunction, you should contact the manufacturer. The device may need to be returned to the manufacturer for service. While AEDs require minimal maintenance, it is important to remember the following:

- Follow the manufacturer's specific recommendations for periodic equipment checks.
- Make sure that the batteries have enough energy for one complete rescue. (A fully charged

LIVING WILLS: A MATTER OF CHOICE

Your 75-year-old grandfather is living with your family. He has a terminal illness and is frequently in the hospital. He has no hope of regaining his health.

One afternoon, you go to his room to give him lunch. As you start to talk to him, you realize he has stopped breathing. You check for signs of life. He has none. You are suddenly faced with the fact that your grandfather is no longer alive. What should you do?

No one but you can answer that question. No one can advise you. No one can predict the outcome of your decision. You alone must decide whether or not to give your grandfather CPR.

Endless questions race through your mind. Can I face the fact I am losing someone I love? Shouldn't I always try to give CPR? What would his life be like after resuscitation? What would grandfather want? Your mind tells you to give CPR, yet your heart tells you not to.

It is important to realize that it is okay to withhold CPR when a terminally ill person is dying. Nature takes its course, and in some cases people feel they have lived full lives and are prepared for death.

Advance Directives

Fortunately, this type of heart-wrenching, last-second decision can sometimes be avoided if loved ones talk to each other in advance about their preferences regarding lifesaving treatments.

Instructions that describe a person's wishes about medical treatment are called *advance directives*. These instructions make known a person's intentions while he or she is still capable of doing so and are used when the person can no longer make his or her own health-care decisions.

As provided by the Federal Patient Self-Determination Act, adults who are admitted to a hospital or a health-care facility or who receive assistance from certain organizations that receive funds from Medicare and Medicaid have the right to make fundamental choices about their own care. They must be told about their right to make decisions about the level of life support that would be provided in an emergency situation. They are supposed to be offered the opportunity to make these choices at the time of admission.

Conversations with relatives, friends or physicians while the patient is still capable of making decisions are the most common form of advance directives. However, because conversations may not be recalled accurately or may not have taken into account the illness or emergency now facing the patient, the courts consider written directives more reliable.

Two examples of written advance directives are *living wills* and *durable powers of attorney for health care*. The types of health-care decisions covered by these docu-

- backup battery should be readily available.)
- Make sure that the correct defibrillator pads are in the package and are properly sealed.
- Check any expiration dates on defibrillation pads and batteries and replace as necessary.
- After use, make sure that all accessories are replaced and that the machine is in proper working order.
- If at any time the machine fails to work properly or warning indicators are recognized, discontinue use and contact the manufacturer immediately.

ments vary by state. Talking with a legal professional can help determine which advance directive options are available in your state and what they cover.

If a person establishes a living will, directions for health care would be in place before he or she became unable to communicate his or her wishes. Instructions that can be included in this document vary from state to state. A living will generally allows a person to refuse only medical care that "merely prolongs the process of dying," such as resuscitating a person with a terminal illness.

If a person has established a durable power of attorney for health care, the document would authorize someone else to make medical decisions for that person in any situation in which the person could no longer make them for him or herself. This authorized person is called a *health-care surrogate* or *proxy*. This surrogate, with the information given by the patient's physician, may consent to or refuse medical treatment on the patient's behalf.

Do Not Resuscitate
A doctor could formalize the person's preferences by writing "Do Not Resuscitate" (DNR) orders in his or her medical records. Such orders would state that if the person's heart or breathing stops, he or she should not be resuscitated. DNR orders may be covered in a living will or in the durable power of attorney for health care.

Appointing someone to act as a health-care surrogate, along with writing down your instructions, is the best way to formalize your wishes about medical care.

Some of these documents can be obtained through a personal physician, attorney or various state and health-care organizations. A lawyer is not always needed to execute advance directives. However, if you have any questions concerning advance directives, it is wise to obtain legal advice.

Talk in Advance
Copies of advance directives should be provided to all personal physicians, family members and the person chosen as the health-care surrogate. Tell them what documents have been prepared and where the original and other copies are located. Discuss the document with all parties so that they understand the intent of all requests. Keep these documents updated.

Keep in mind that advance directives are not limited to elderly people or people with terminal illnesses. Advance directives should be considered by anyone who has decided on the care he or she would like to have provided. An unexpected illness or injury could create a need for decisions at any time.

Knowing about living wills, durable powers of attorney for health care and DNR orders can help you prepare for difficult decisions. If you are interested in learning more about your rights and the options available to you in your state, contact a legal professional.

REFERENCES
1. Hospital Shared Services of Colorado, Stockard Inventory Program. Your Right to Make Health Care Decisions. Denver, Colorado, 1991.
2. Title 42 United States Code Section 1395 cc (a)(1)(Q)(A).Patient Self-Determination Act.

CPR—Adult

After checking an ill or injured person

STEP 1

Give cycles of **30** chest compressions and **2** rescue breaths.

STEP 2

Continue CPR until—

- Scene becomes unsafe.
- You find a sign of life.
- AED is ready to use.
- You are too exhausted to continue.
- Another trained responder arrives and takes over.

WHAT TO DO NEXT

USE AN AED AS SOON AS ONE BECOMES AVAILABLE

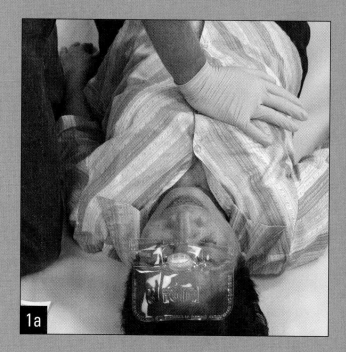

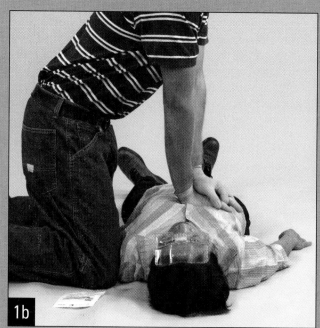

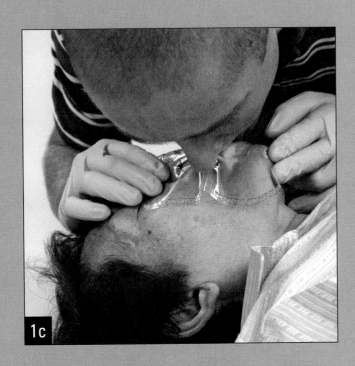

Unconscious Choking—Adult

(BREATHS DO NOT GO IN)

After checking an ill or injured person

STEP 1

Tilt head farther back.
Try **2** rescue breaths again.

STEP 2

If chest does not rise—
Give **30** chest compressions.

*(**TIP:** Remove breathing barrier when giving chest compressions.)*

STEP 3

Look for an object.

STEP 4

Remove if one is seen.

STEP 5

Try **2** rescue breaths.

WHAT TO DO NEXT

IF BREATHS DO NOT GO IN—
Continue Steps 2-5.

IF BREATHS GO IN—
  • Check for signs of life.
  • Give care based on conditions found.

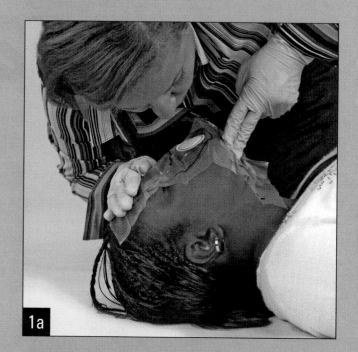

1a

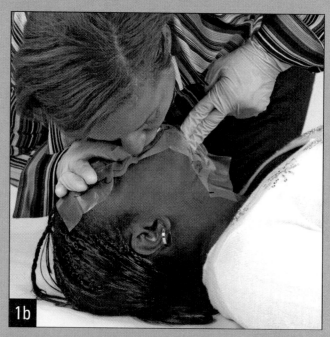

1b

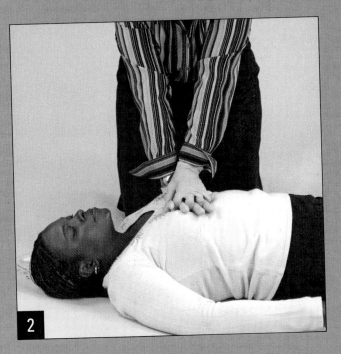

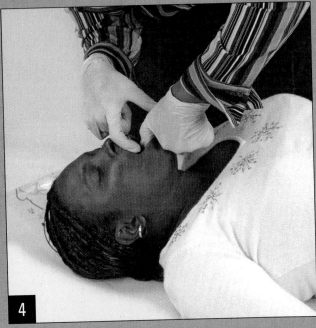

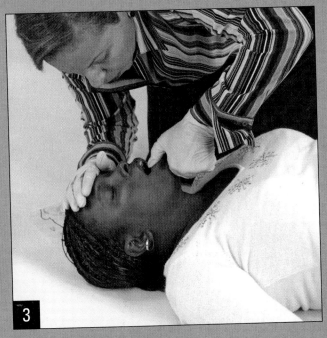

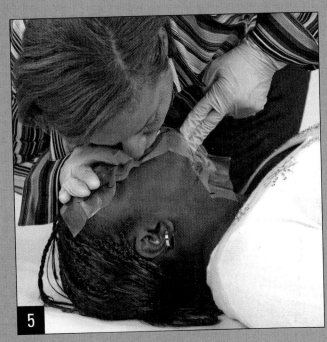

CPR—Child

After checking an ill or injured child

STEP 1

Give cycles of **30** chest compressions and **2** rescue breaths.

STEP 2

Continue CPR until—

- Scene becomes unsafe.
- You find a sign of life.
- AED is ready to use.
- You are too exhausted to continue.
- Another trained responder arrives and takes over.

WHAT TO DO NEXT

IF AN AED BECOMES AVAILABLE, Use an AED. IF PULSE, BUT NO BREATHING, Give rescue breathing.

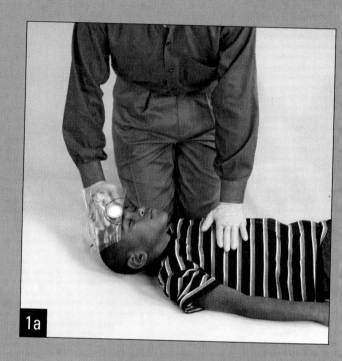

1a

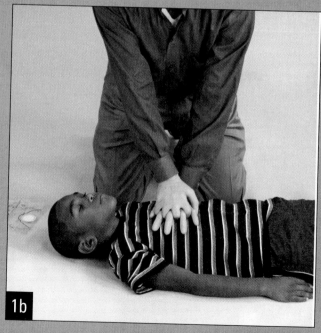

1b

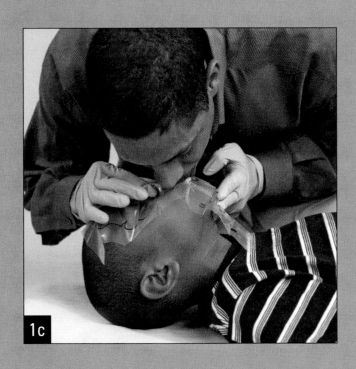

Unconscious Choking—Child

After checking an ill or injured child

STEP 1

Retilt child's head.
Try **2** rescue breaths again.

STEP 2

If chest does not rise—
Give **30** chest compressions.

(TIP: Remove breathing barrier when giving chest compressions.)

STEP 3

Look for an object.

STEP 4

Remove if one is seen.

STEP 5

Try **2** rescue breaths.

WHAT TO DO NEXT

IF BREATHS DO NOT GO IN—
Continue Steps 2-5.

IF BREATHS GO IN—
- Check for signs of life including a pulse.
- Give care based on conditions found.

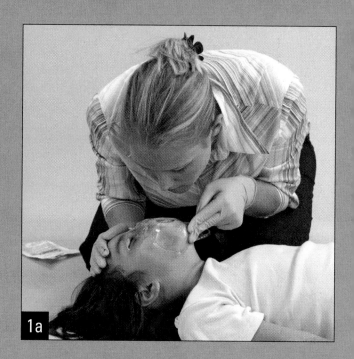

1a

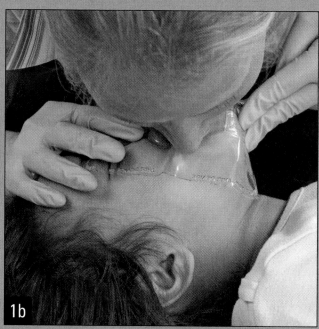

1b

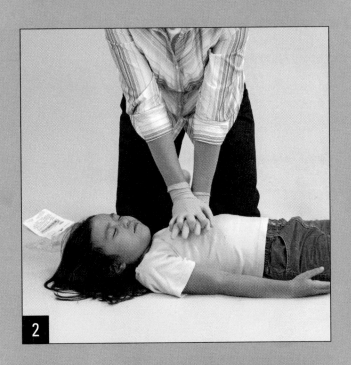

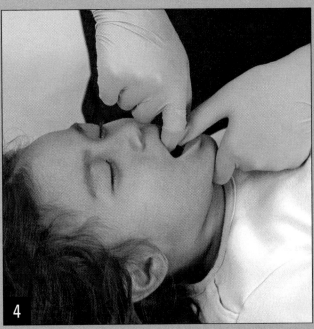

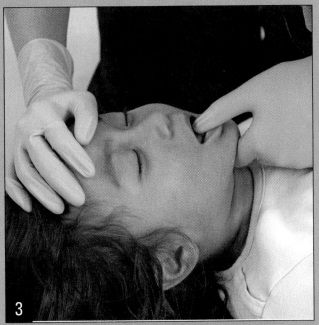

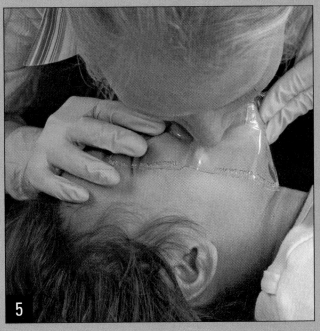

CPR—Infant

After checking an ill or injured infant

STEP 1

Give cycles of **30** chest compressions and **2** rescue breaths.

STEP 2

Continue CPR until—

- Scene becomes unsafe.
- You find signs of life.
- You are too exhausted to continue.
- Another trained responder arrives and takes over.

WHAT TO DO NEXT

IF NO SIGNS OF LIFE—Continue CPR.

IF A PULSE, BUT NO BREATHING—
Give rescue breathing.

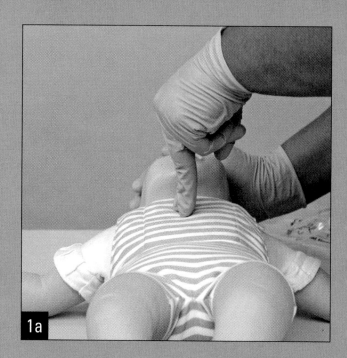

1a

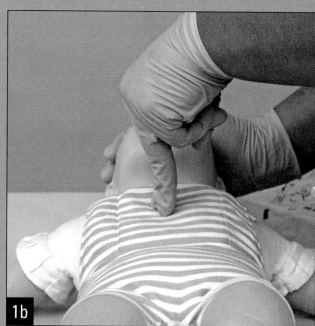

1b

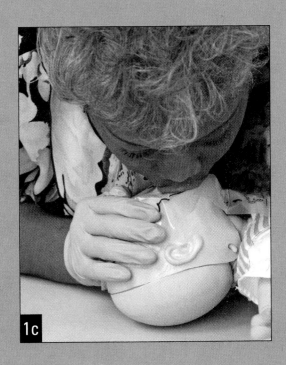

Unconscious Choking—Infant

(BREATHS DO NOT GO IN)

After checking an ill or injured infant

STEP 1

Retilt infant's head.
Try **2** rescue breaths again.

STEP 2

If chest does not rise—
Give **30** chest compressions.

> *(**TIP:** Remove breathing barrier when giving chest compressions.)*

STEP 3

Look for an object.

STEP 4

Remove if one is seen.

STEP 5

Try **2** rescue breaths.

WHAT TO DO NEXT

IF BREATHS DO NOT GO IN—
Continue Steps 2-5.

IF BREATHS GO IN—
- Check for signs of life including a pulse.
- Give care based on conditions found.

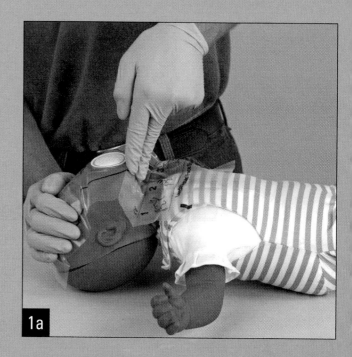

1a

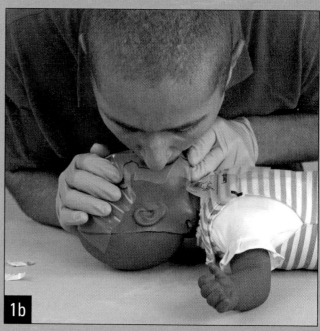

1b

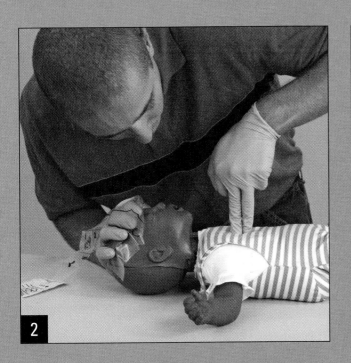

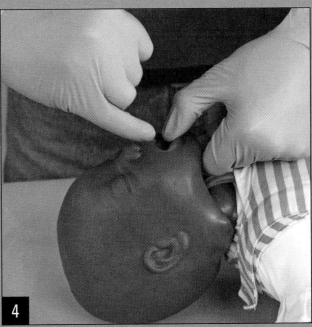

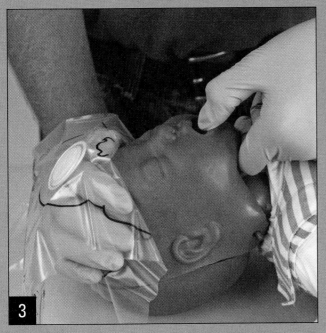

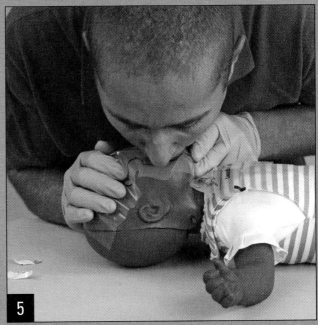

AED—Adult

(NOTE: If two trained responders are present, one should perform CPR while the second responder operates the AED.)

(NO SIGNS OF LIFE) (OVER AGE 8 OR MORE THAN 55 POUNDS)

After checking an ill or injured person

STEP 1
Turn on AED.

STEP 2
Wipe chest dry.

*(**NOTE:** Remove any medication patches with a gloved hand.)*

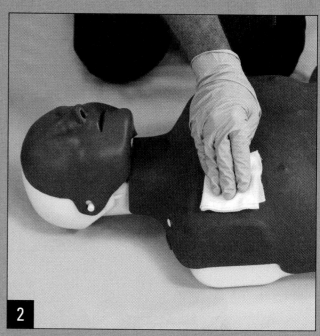

STEP 3
Attach pads to bare chest.

STEP 4
Plug in connector, if necessary.

STEP 5
- Make sure no one, including you, is touching the person.
- Say, "EVERYONE STAND CLEAR."

STEP 6
Push "analyze" button, if necessary. Let AED analyze heart rhythm.

STEP 7
IF SHOCK ADVISED—
- Make sure no one, including you, is touching the person.
- Say, "EVERYONE STAND CLEAR."
- Push "shock" button, if necessary.

WHAT TO DO NEXT
After shock—Give **5** cycles or about **2** minutes of CPR. Let AED reanalyze.

IF NO SHOCK ADVISED—Give **5** cycles or about **2** minutes of CPR.

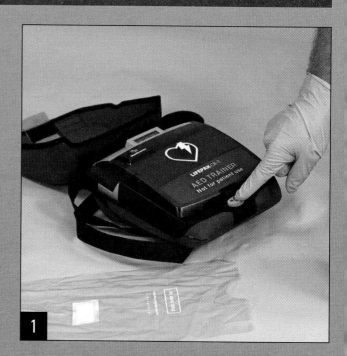

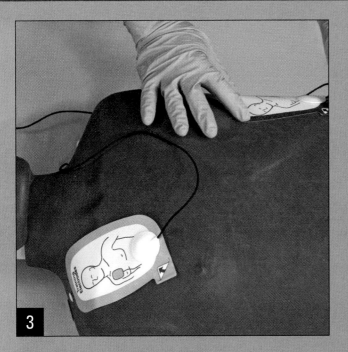

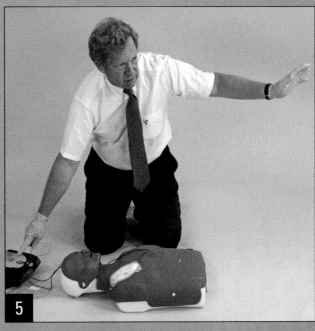

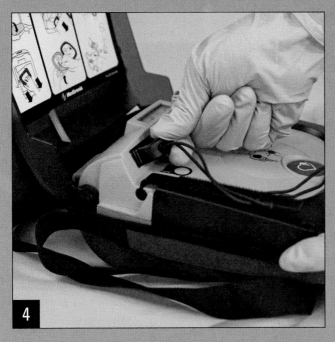

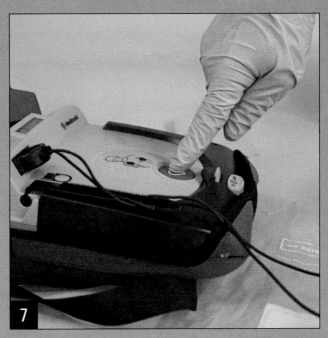

AED—Child

> (**NOTE:** If two trained responders are present, one should perform CPR while the second responder operates the AED.)

(NO SIGNS OF LIFE AND NO PULSE)

After checking an ill or injured child
For Child (ages 1-8 or less than 55 pounds)

STEP 1
Turn on AED.

STEP 2
Wipe chest dry.

STEP 3
Attach **pediatric pads** to bare chest.
- If pads risk touching each other, use front/back pad placement.

STEP 4
Plug in connector, if necessary.

STEP 5
- Make sure no one, including you, is touching the child.
- Say, "EVERYONE STAND CLEAR."

STEP 6
Push "analyze" button, if necessary. Let the AED analyze the heart rhythm.

STEP 7
IF SHOCK ADVISED—
- Make sure no one, including you, is touching the child.
- Say, "EVERYONE STAND CLEAR."
- Push "shock" button, if necessary.

WHAT TO DO NEXT
After shock—Give **5** cycles or about **2** minutes of CPR. Let AED reanalyze.

IF NO SHOCK ADVISED—Give **5** cycles or about **2** minutes of CPR.

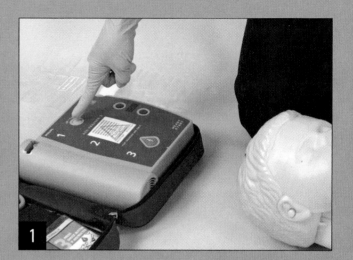

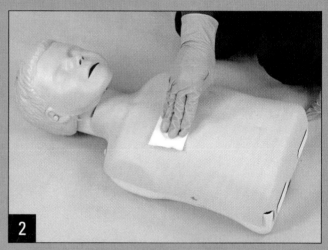

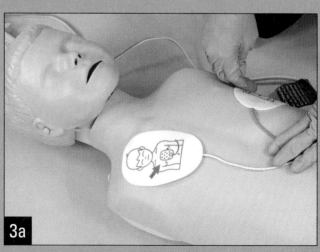

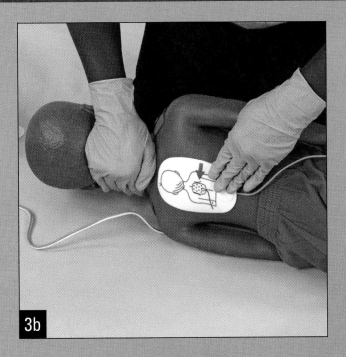

3b

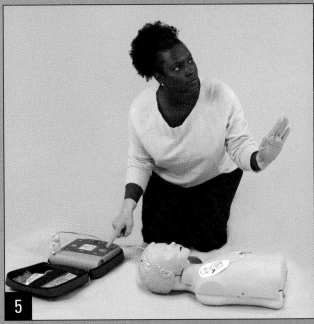

5

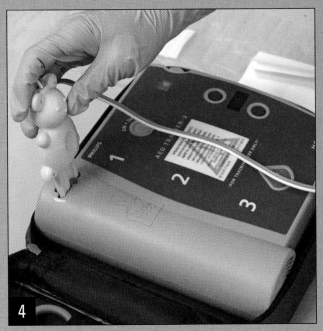

4

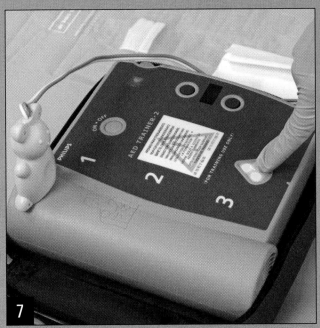

7

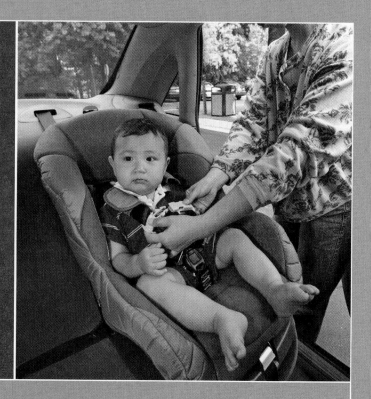

6

Injuries and illness cost billions of dollars each year in lost wages, medical expenses, insurance, property damage and other indirect costs.

Chapter 6

Injury Prevention

The wail of sirens breaks the sleepy afternoon stillness of the shady street. A police car suddenly pulls to a stop in front of a house. An ambulance drives up and two paramedics dart into the house. Another ambulance quickly arrives. For a few moments, all is quiet. Suddenly several people emerge from the house carrying a stretcher. On it is a small body. Paramedics cluster around, frantically trying to save the child's life. They slide the stretcher into the ambulance. A distraught woman runs after them. She turns to the police officer next to her. "She was just playing on the bed," she chokes. "She must have fallen off the side...."

Injuries and illness cost billions of dollars each year in lost wages, medical expenses, insurance, property damage and other indirect costs. But illness and injury are not simply unpleasant facts of life to be shrugged off as inevitable. Often you can prevent them by taking safety precautions and choosing a lifestyle that promotes optimal health.

INJURIES

Each year in the United States an estimated one in 12 people requires medical treatment for an injury. An estimated 170,000 people die from the injuries they receive. Injury is the leading cause of death for people of all ages (Fig. 6-1).

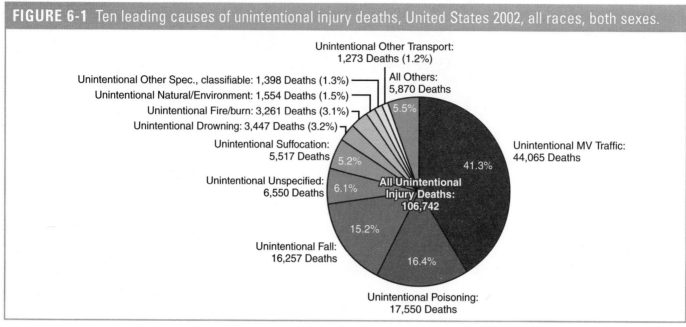

Unintentional Other Transport:
1,273 Deaths (1.2%)

Unintentional Other Spec., classifiable: 1,398 Deaths (1.3%)
Unintentional Natural/Environment: 1,554 Deaths (1.5%)
Unintentional Fire/burn: 3,261 Deaths (3.1%)
Unintentional Drowning: 3,447 Deaths (3.2%)
Unintentional Suffocation:
5,517 Deaths

Unintentional Unspecified:
6,550 Deaths

Unintentional Fall:
16,257 Deaths

All Others:
5,870 Deaths

5.5%

Unintentional MV Traffic:
44,065 Deaths

41.3%

All Unintentional
Injury Deaths:
106,742

5.2%

6.1%

15.2%

16.4%

Unintentional Poisoning:
17,550 Deaths

Data Source: National Center for Health Statistics (NCHS), National Vital Statistics System. *www.cdc.gov/ncipc/wisgars/default.htm* Accessed 11/15/05.

Injury Risk Factors

A number of factors affect a person's risk of being injured—age, gender, geographic location, economic status and alcohol use and abuse. Technology also affects the type and frequency of injury. As certain activities, such as skateboarding and rollerblading, gain and lose popularity, injury statistics reflect the changes.

- Injury rates are highest among people younger than age 39. People ages 15 to 24 and people ages 65 and older have the highest rate of deaths from injury.
- Gender is also a significant factor in risk of injury. Males are at greater risk than females for any type of injury. In general, men are about twice as likely to suffer a fatal injury as women.
- Many environmental factors influence injury rates. Whether you live on a farm or in the city, whether your home is built out of wood or brick, the type of heat used in your home and your local climate all affect your degree of risk. For instance, death rates from

injury are higher in rural areas. The death rate from injuries is twice as high in low-income areas as it is in high-income areas.

- Alcohol use and abuse is a significant factor in many injuries and fatalities, even in teenagers. In 2002, approximately 17,500 people in the United States died in alcohol-related motor vehicle crashes. This figure accounts for 41 percent of all traffic-related deaths. It is also estimated that a significant number of victims who die as a result of falls, drownings, fires, assaults and suicides have blood alcohol concentrations over the legal limit.

Reducing Your Risk of Injury

Despite the statistics showing that people of certain ages and gender are injured more often than others, your chances of injury have more to do with what you do than who you are. Injuries do not just happen. Many injuries are preventable, predictable events resulting from the way people interact with the potential dangers in the environ-

ment. The following are general strategies for preventing injuries:

- Encourage or persuade people at risk to change their behavior.
- Require people at risk to change their behavior, such as mandatory safety belt laws.
- Provide products that offer automatic protection, such as air bags, designed to reduce the risk of injury.

In addition, you can reduce your own risk of an injury by taking the following steps:

- **Know your risk.**
- **Take measures that make a difference.** Change behaviors that increase your risk of injury and risk injuring others.
- **Think safety.** Be alert for and avoid potentially harmful conditions or activities that increase your injury risk. Take precautions, such as wearing appropriate protective devices—helmets, padding and eyewear—and buckle up when driving or riding in motor vehicles.
- **Learn and use first aid skills.** Despite dramatic improvements in

emergency medical systems nationwide over the past decade, the person who can often make the difference between life and death is you, when you apply your first aid training.

Vehicle Safety. When riding in a motor vehicle, buckle up. Although more cars than ever are equipped with airbags, wearing a safety belt is the easiest and best action you can take to prevent injury in a motor-vehicle collision. Always wear a safety belt including a shoulder restraint when riding in the front or back seats. In most states, wearing a safety belt is required by law. In 2002, safety belts saved more than 13,000 lives.

The economic burden of motor vehicle-related deaths and injuries is also enormous, costing the United States more than $150 billion each year. More than 41,000 people in the United States die in motor vehicle crashes each year, and crash injuries result in about 500,000 hospitalizations and 4 million emergency department visits annually.

Infants and children should always ride in approved safety seats in the back seat (Fig. 6-2). Infants under 1 year of age and weighing less than 20 pounds should ride in a safety seat facing the rear of the vehicle to protect the infant's head and neck. Children between the ages of 4 and 8 should use a booster seat so the safety belt fits correctly, and ride in a middle or back seat. Although airbags have saved many lives, they also pose several risks to children. The amount of force during airbag deployment can kill or severely injure children occupying the front seat. Always have children under the age of 13 years sit in the rear, away from airbags.

For children, motor-vehicle crashes are the major cause of death as a result of injury. All 50 states and the District of Columbia require the

FIGURE 6-2 Infants and children should always ride in approved safety seats.

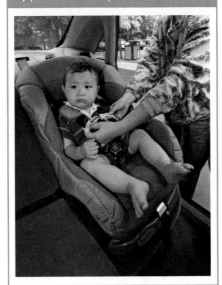

use of child safety seats. Unsecured toys and other objects can turn into high-speed missiles in a vehicle crash. Do not leave objects loose in your vehicle.

Do not drink and drive. Plan ahead to find a ride or take a cab or public transportation if you are going to a party where you may drink alcohol. If you are with a group, designate a driver who agrees not to drink on this occasion. Do not drink if you are in a boat. The U.S. Coast Guard reports that more than 50 percent of drownings from boating incidents involve alcohol.

Fire Safety. Nearly 3400 people died in residential fires in the United States in 2002. In nearly two-thirds of these fires, smoke alarms were either missing or not working properly. Regardless of the cause of fires, everyone needs to know how to respond in case of fire:

- Install a smoke alarm on every floor of your home. Check the batteries once a month, and change

the batteries at least twice a year.
- Keep fire extinguishers where they are most likely to be needed and keep matches out of children's reach.
- Always keep space heaters away from curtains and other flammable materials.
- Install guards around fireplaces, radiators, pipes and woodburning stoves.
- Set your water temperature at 120° F or less to prevent scalding from tap water in sinks and bathtubs.

- Cook on back burners when possible and always turn pot handles toward the back of the stove.
- Keep highchairs away from the stove and other hot appliances and cribs away from radiators and other hot surfaces.
- Keep hot liquids and foods out of children's reach.
- Test the temperature of heated food before serving it to a child.
- Plan and practice a fire escape route with your family or room-mates (Fig. 6-3).
  - Gather everyone together at a convenient time.
  - Sketch a floor plan of all rooms, including doors, windows and hallways. Include all floors of the home.
  - Plan and draw the escape plan with arrows showing two ways, if possible, to get out of each room. Sleeping areas are most important, since many fires happen at night.
    - Plan to use stairs only, never an elevator.
    - Plan where everyone will meet after leaving the building.
  - Designate who should call the fire department and from which phone.
    - Plan to leave the burning building first and then call from a phone nearby, if possible.

Remember and use the following guidelines to escape from fire:

- If smoke is present, crawl low to escape. Because smoke rises in a fire, breathable air is often close to the floor.
- Make sure children can open windows, go down a ladder and lower themselves to the ground. Practice with them. Always lower

FIGURE 6-3 Plan a fire escape route for your home.

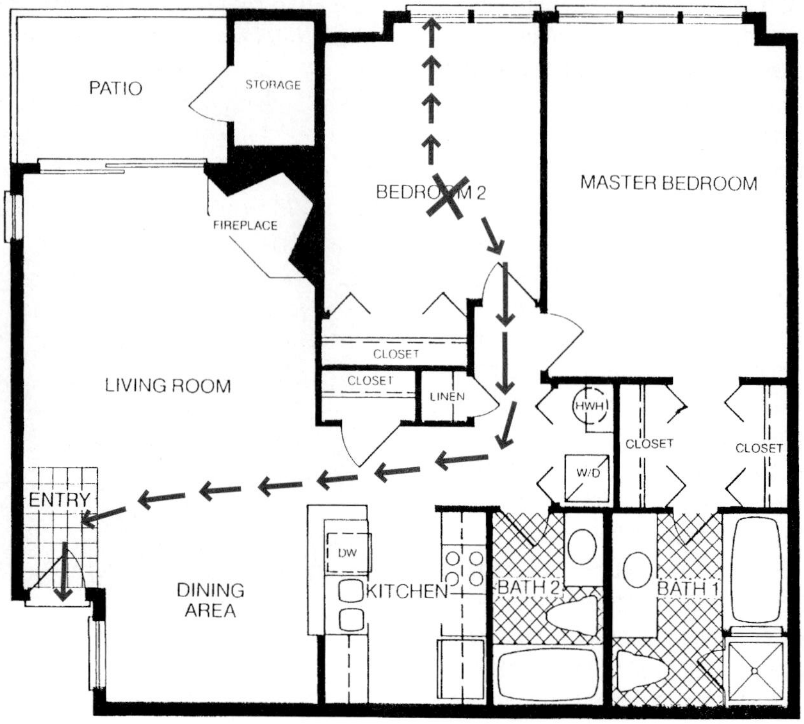

children to the ground first before you go out a window.
- Get out quickly and do not, under any circumstances, return to a burning building.
- If you cannot escape, stay in the room and stuff door cracks and vents with wet towels, rags or clothing. If a phone is available, call the fire department—even if rescuers are already outside—and tell the call taker your location.

Contact your local fire department for additional safety guidelines.

Safety at Home. About 8 million disabling injuries occur in homes each year in the United States. The three leading causes of accidental death in the home are poisoning, falls and fire. Most falls occur around the home. Young children and the elderly are fre-

quent victims of falls. Removing hazards and practicing good safety habits will make your home safer. You can get a good start on this by making a list of the needed improvements. Safety at home is relatively simple and relies largely on common sense. Taking the following steps will help make your home a safer place:

- Post emergency numbers—9-1-1 or the local emergency number, Poison Control Center (800-222-1222), physician, as well as other important numbers—near every phone.
- Make sure that stairways and hallways are well lit.
- Equip stairways with handrails, and use nonslip treads or securely fastened rugs.
- Secure rugs to the floor with double-sided tape.

- If moisture accumulates in damp spots, correct the cause of the problem. Clean up spills promptly.
- Keep medicines and poisonous substances separate from each other and from food. They should be out of reach of children and in secured cabinets.
- Keep medicines in their original containers with safety caps.
- Keep your heating and cooling systems and all appliances in good working order. Check heating and cooling systems annually before use.
- Read and follow manufacturers' instructions for electrical tools, appliances and toys.
- Turn off the oven and other appliances when not using them. Unplug certain appliances, such as an iron, curling iron, coffeemaker or portable heater, after each use.
- Make sure that your home has at least one working, easily accessible fire extinguisher and everyone knows how to use it.
- Keep firearms unloaded in a locked place, out of the reach of children and stored separately from ammunition.
- Practice safe firearms storage, handling and education.
- Try crawling around your home to see it as an infant or young child sees it. You may become aware of unsuspected hazards.
- Ensure that cords for lamps and other items are not placed where someone can trip over them.

This list does not include all the safety measures you need to take in your home. If young children or elderly or ill individuals live with you, you will need to take additional steps, depending upon the individual characteristics of your home.

For an elderly person, you may need to install handrails in the bathtub or shower and beside the toilet. You may need a bath chair or bench. Always have a mat with a suction base if your tub does not have nonslip strips built in. A safe bath water temperature is 101° F (38° C).

Safety at Work. Most people spend approximately one-third of their day at work. To improve safety at work, you should be aware of the following:

- Fire evacuation procedures
- How to activate your emergency response team and how to call 9-1-1 or the local emergency number
- Location of the nearest fire extinguisher and first aid kit
- Use recommended safety equipment and follow safety procedures if you work in an environment where hazards exist
- Workplace safety training

Safety at Play. Make sports and other recreational activities safe by always following accepted guidelines for the activity.

Bike Safety. Each year, approximately 500,000 people are non-fatally injured while riding a bicycle. Ninety percent of bicyclists killed in 2000 reportedly were not wearing helmets. When cycling, always wear an approved helmet. The head or neck is the most seriously injured part of the body in most fatally injured cyclists. Children should wear a helmet even if they are still riding along the sidewalk on training wheels. Some states have helmet laws that apply to young children.

Look for a helmet approved by the Snell Memorial Foundation or the American National Standards Institute (ANSI), and make sure the helmet is the correct size and that it fits comfortably and securely. Keep off roads that are busy or have no shoulder. Wear

reflective clothing, and make sure you have a headlight, taillight and reflectors on your bicycle wheels if you cycle at night. Make sure your bicycle and your child's bicycle are in good condition. Most bicycle mishaps happen within a mile of home.

Eye and Foot Safety. With any activity in which eyes could be injured, such as racquetball, wear protective goggles.

Appropriate footwear is also important in preventing injuries. For activities involving physical contact, wear properly fitted protective equipment to avoid serious injury. Above all, know and follow the rules of the sport.

Swimming, Water and Running Safety. If you do not know how to swim, learn how or always wear an appropriate flotation device if you are going to be in, on or around the water. Many people who drown never intended to be in the water at all. Be careful when walking beside rivers, lakes and other bodies of water. Dangerous undercurrents in shallow water can catch even the best of swimmers.

If you or a family member don't know how to swim, or would like to improve your swimming skills, contact your local American Red Cross chapter to sign up for a Red Cross swimming and water safety class.

To prevent water-related injuries, you should also—

- Always closely supervise children in, on or near water. Stay within arm's reach of them.
- If you have a backyard pool, make sure it is separated from your home's entrance by a fence. The fence should completely enclose the pool and be designed so that children cannot easily climb over it. The fence should be equipped with a self-closing,

self-latching gate that cannot be easily opened by a young child.

- Cover wading pools when not in use.
- Keep toilet seat lids down when the toilet is not being used.
- Never drink alcohol while you drive a boat and do not travel in a boat operated by a driver who has been drinking.

If you run, jog or walk, plan your route carefully. Exercise only in well-lit, well-populated areas, and consider exercising with another person. Keep off busy roads. If you must exercise outdoors after dark, wear reflective clothing and move facing traffic. Be alert for cars pulling out at intersections and driveways.

Whenever you start an activity unfamiliar to you, such as boating, skiing or motorcycle riding, take lessons to learn how to do the sport safely. Many mishaps result from inexperience. Make sure your equipment is in good working order.

INJURY PREVENTION SURVEY

Injuries do not just happen. For the most part, they are predictable and preventable. This survey will help make you more aware of conditions or situations around you that may lead to injury. It also may help you reduce your risk of injury, as well as your risk to others.

Mark "Yes" or "No" next to the following questions:

Yes	No	
☑	☐	Do you wear a safety belt when driving or riding in a motor vehicle?
☑	☐	Do you refrain from driving after drinking alcoholic beverages?
☑	☐	Do the stairs where you work have handrails?
☑	☐	Do you use a stepladder or sturdy stool to reach high, out-of-reach objects?
☑	☐	Do you have adequate lighting in halls and stairways?
☐	☑	Do you use good lifting techniques when lifting objects?
☑	☐	Do you wear an appropriate helmet when using a bicycle, motorcycle or scooter?
☑	☐	Do you wear a lifejacket on or around the water?
☑	☐	Do you wear safety protection (e.g., goggles and hearing protection) and follow equipment safety recommendations when operating power tools?

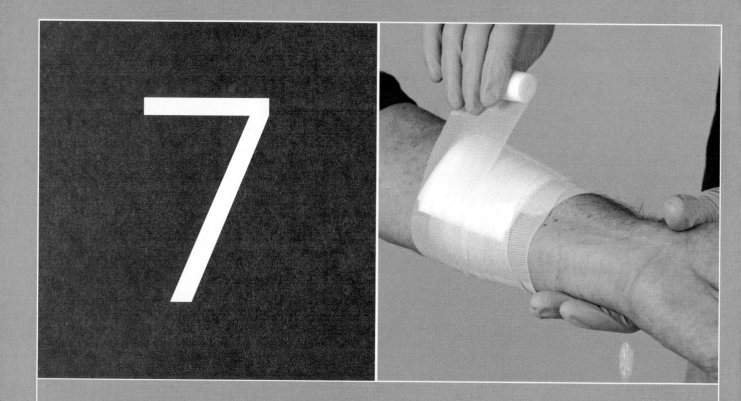

7

Any time the soft tissues are damaged or torn, the body is threatened.

Chapter 7

Soft Tissue Injuries: Cuts, Scrapes and Bruises

An infant falls and bruises his arm while learning to walk. A toddler scrapes her knee while learning to run. A child falls off the monkeybars and needs stitches. A teenager bruises a leg playing basketball. A college student suffers sunburn during a weekend at the beach. An adult cuts his hand while working in a woodshop. What do all these injuries have in common? They are all soft tissue injuries.

Soft tissues are the layers of skin and the fat and muscle beneath the skin's outer layer (Fig. 7-1). Any time the soft tissues are damaged or torn, the body is threatened. Injuries may damage the soft tissues at or near the skin's surface or deep in the body. Severe bleeding can occur at the skin's surface and under it, where it is harder to detect. Germs can get into the body through a scrape, cut or puncture and cause infection.

Burns are a special kind of soft tissue injury. Like other types of soft tissue injury, burns can damage the top layer of skin or the skin and the layers of fat, muscle and bone beneath.

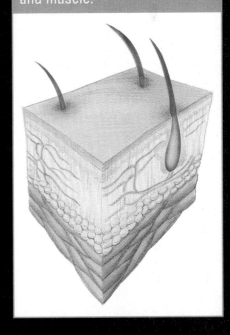

FIGURE 7-1 The soft tissues include the layers of skin, fat and muscle.

WOUNDS

An injury to the soft tissues is commonly called a wound. Wounds are usually classified as either closed or open. In a closed wound, the skin's surface is not broken and the damage happens below the surface, where bleeding sometimes occurs. In an open wound, the skin's surface is broken and blood may come through the tear in the skin.

Fortunately, most of the bleeding you will encounter will not be serious. It will usually stop by itself within a few minutes, with minimal intervention. The wound will cause a blood vessel to tear, but the blood at the wound will soon clot and stop flowing. Sometimes, however, the damaged blood vessel will be too large or the pressure in the blood vessel too great for the blood to clot. Then bleeding can be life threatening. This can happen with both closed and open wounds.

CRITICAL FACTS

SIGNALS OF INTERNAL BLEEDING

- Tender, swollen, bruised or hard areas of the body, such as the abdomen
- Rapid, weak pulse
- Skin that feels cool or moist or looks pale or bluish
- Vomiting blood or coughing up blood
- Excessive thirst
- Becoming confused, faint, drowsy or unconscious

Closed Wounds

The simplest closed wound is a bruise, which develops when the body is bumped or hit, such as when you bump your leg on a table or chair (Fig. 7-2). The force of the blow to the body damages the soft tissue layers beneath the skin, causing internal bleeding. Blood and other fluids seep into the surrounding tissues, causing the area to swell and change color.

A much more serious closed wound can be caused by a violent force hitting the body. This type of force can injure larger blood vessels and deeper layers of muscle tissue, causing heavy bleeding beneath the skin.

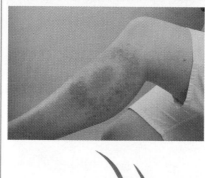

FIGURE 7-2 The simplest closed wound is a bruise, which develops when the body is bumped or hit.

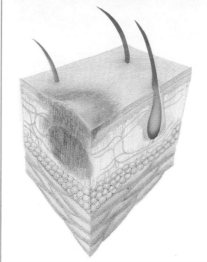

Caring for Closed Wounds.

Many closed wounds, like bruises, do not require special medical care. To care for a closed wound, you can apply direct pressure on the area to decrease bleeding beneath the skin, as long as you keep the injured area still. Applying cold can be effective early on in helping control both pain and swelling (Fig. 7-3). Fill a plastic bag with ice or wrap ice with a damp cloth and apply it to the injured area for periods of about 20 minutes. Place a thin barrier between the ice and bare skin. Remove the ice for 20 minutes before applying it again. Elevating the injured part may help reduce swelling. However, *do not* elevate the injured part if it causes more pain.

Do not assume that all closed wounds are minor injuries. Take the time to find out whether more serious injuries could be present. Call 9-1-1 or the local emergency number if—

- A person complains of severe pain or cannot move a body part without pain.
- You think the force that caused the injury was great enough to cause serious damage.
- An injured extremity is blue or extremely pale.

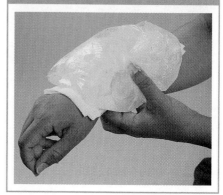

FIGURE 7-3 Apply ice to a closed wound to help control pain and swelling.

In these cases, the person may be bleeding internally and need emergency medical help as soon as possible.

With all closed wounds, help the person rest in the most comfortable position, keep the person from getting chilled or overheated, and reassure and comfort the person. Be sure that a person with an injured lower extremity does not bear weight until advised by a medical professional.

Open Wounds

In an open wound, the break in the skin can be as minor as a scrape of the surface layers or as severe as a deep penetration. The amount of bleeding depends on the location and severity of the injury.

The four main types of open wounds are—

- **Abrasions.** These are the most common type of open wound (Fig. 7-4). They are often caused by something rubbing roughly against the skin. Abrasions do not bleed very much and the bleeding they do cause comes from capillaries (tiny blood vessels). Because dirt and germs are frequently rubbed into this type of wound, it is important to clean it thoroughly with soap and water to prevent infection. An abrasion is sometimes called a scrape, a rug burn, a road rash or a strawberry. An abrasion is usually painful because scraping of the outer skin layers exposes sensitive nerve endings.

FIGURE 7-4 Abrasion.

INFECTION

When an injury breaks the skin, the best initial defense against infection is to clean the area. For minor wounds, wash the area with soap and water. Most soaps are effective in removing harmful bacteria. You do not need to wash wounds that require medical attention because they involve more extensive tissue damage or bleeding. It is more important to control the bleeding.

Because infected wounds can cause serious medical problems, it is important to maintain an up-to-date immunization record. Immunizations help your body fight infection. One of these immunizations prevents tetanus, a serious disease. The best way to prevent tetanus is to receive a booster shot from your health-care provider every 10 years, because the protective effect of the vaccine decreases over time.

Sometimes, even the best care for a soft tissue injury is not enough to prevent infection. You will usually be able to recognize the early signals of infection. The area around the wound becomes swollen and red. The area may feel warm or throb with pain. Some wounds discharge pus. Serious infections may cause a person to develop a fever and feel ill. Red streaks may develop that progress from the wound in the direction of the heart. If this happens, the infected person should seek immediate professional medical attention.

If you see any signals of infection, keep the area clean, soak it in warm water and apply a triple-antibiotic ointment if the person has no known allergies or sensitivities to the medication. Change coverings over the wound daily.

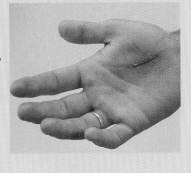

- **Lacerations.** A laceration is a cut in the skin and is commonly caused by a sharp object, such as a knife, scissors or broken glass (Fig. 7-5). A laceration also can happen when a blunt force splits the skin. Deep lacerations can cut layers of fat and muscle, damaging both nerves and blood vessels. Lacerations can bleed heavily but may also not bleed at all. Lacerations are not always painful because damaged nerves cannot send pain signals to the brain. Lacerations can easily become infected if not cared for properly.
- **Avulsions.** An avulsion is an injury in which a portion of the skin and sometimes other soft tissue is partially or completely torn away (Fig. 7-6). A violent force may completely tear away a body part (i.e., amputation) such as a finger. Because an avulsion often damages deeper tissues, bleeding is often significant. In contrast, when a body part is completely torn away, bleeding is easier to control because the tissues close around the vessels at the injury site.
- **Punctures.** Punctures are usually caused by a pointed object, such as a nail, piercing the skin (Fig. 7-7). A gunshot wound is also a puncture wound. Punctures do not bleed very much unless a blood vessel has been injured. However, an object that goes into the soft tissues beneath the skin can carry germs deep into the body. These germs can cause infections—sometimes serious ones. If the object remains in the wound, it is called an *embedded object*.

Caring for Open Wounds. All open wounds need some type of covering to help control bleeding and prevent infection. These coverings are commonly referred to as dressings and bandages, and there are many types.

Dressings are pads placed directly on the wound to absorb blood and other fluids and to prevent infection. To minimize the chance of infection, dressings should be sterile. Most dressings are porous, allowing air to circulate to the wound to promote healing. Standard dressings include varying sizes of cotton gauze, commonly ranging from 2 to 4 inches square. Much larger dressings are used to cover very large wounds and multiple wounds in one body area. Some dressings have nonstick surfaces to prevent them from sticking to the wound (Fig. 7-8).

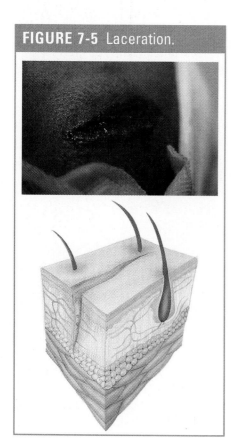

FIGURE 7-5 Laceration.

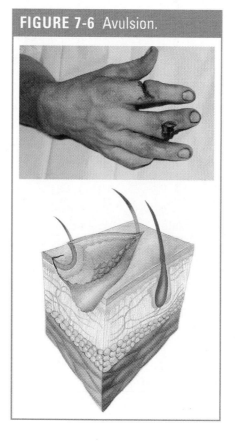

FIGURE 7-6 Avulsion.

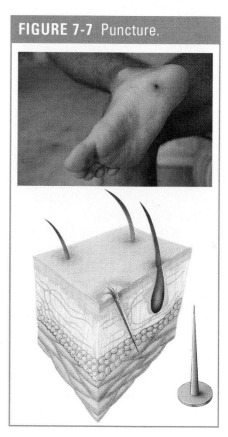

FIGURE 7-7 Puncture.

An *occlusive dressing* is a bandage or dressing that closes a wound or damaged area of the body and prevents it from being exposed to the air (Fig. 7-9). By preventing exposure to the air, occlusive dressings help prevent infection. Occlusive dressings help keep in medications that are applied to the affected area. They also help keep in heat, body fluids and moisture. Occlusive dressing comes from the Latin word "occludere," meaning "to close up," and the Old French word "dresser," meaning "to arrange." Put the words together and you have "to arrange to close up." An example of an occlusive dressing is plastic wrap. This type of dressing is used for certain chest and abdominal injuries.

Bandages. A *bandage* is any material that is used to wrap or cover any part of the body. Bandages are used to hold dressings in place, to apply pressure to control bleeding, to protect a wound from dirt and infection and to provide support to an injured limb or body part (Fig. 7-10). Any bandage applied snugly to create pressure on a wound or an injury is called a *pressure bandage*.

You can purchase many different types of bandages, including—

- *Adhesive compresses*, which are available in assorted sizes and consist of a small pad of nonstick gauze on a strip of adhesive tape that is applied directly to minor wounds (Fig. 7-11).
- *Bandage compresses*, which are thick gauze dressings attached to a bandage that is tied in place. Bandage compresses are specially designed to help control severe bleeding and usually come in sterile packages.
- *Roller bandages*, which are usually made of gauze or gauze-like material (Fig. 7-12). Roller bandages are available in assorted widths from ½ to 12 inches (1.3 to 30.5 centimeters) and lengths from 5 to 10 yards

FIGURE 7-8 Dressings are placed directly on the wound to absorb blood and prevent infection.

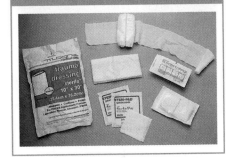

FIGURE 7-9 Occlusive dressings are designed to prevent air from passing through.

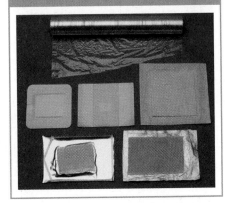

FIGURE 7-10 Bandages are used to hold dressings in place, control bleeding, protect wounds and provide support to an injured limb or body part.

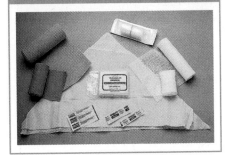

TETANUS

Tetanus is a severe infection that can result from a puncture or a deep cut. Tetanus is a disease caused by bacteria that produces a powerful poison in the body. The poison enters the nervous system and can cause muscle paralysis. Once tetanus reaches the nervous system, its effects are highly dangerous and can be fatal. Fortunately, tetanus often can be successfully treated with medicines called *antitoxins.*

One way to prevent tetanus is through immunizations. We all need to have a shot that protects us against tetanus, and a booster shot at least every 10 years. Anyone whose skin is punctured or who is cut by an object that can carry infection, such as a rusty nail, or is bitten by an animal should check with his or her health-care provider to learn whether a booster shot is needed.

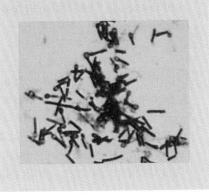

FIGURE 7-11 Adhesive compress.

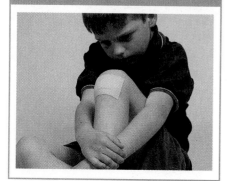

FIGURE 7-12 Roller bandage.

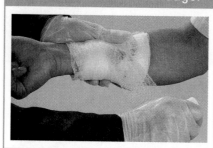

(4.6 to 9.1 meters). A narrow bandage would be used to wrap a hand or wrist. A medium-width bandage would be used for an arm or ankle. A wide bandage would be used to wrap a leg. A roller bandage is generally wrapped around the body part. It can be tied or taped in place. A roller bandage may also be used to hold a dressing in place, secure a splint or control external bleeding.

Follow these general guidelines when applying a roller bandage:

- Check for feeling, warmth and color of the area below the injury site, especially fingers and toes, before and after applying the bandage.
- Elevate the injured body part if you do not suspect a broken bone and it does not cause more pain.
- Secure the end of the bandage in place with a turn of the bandage. Wrap the bandage around the body part until the dressing is completely covered and the bandage extends several inches beyond the dressing. Tie or tape the bandage in place (Fig. 7-13, A-C).
- Do not cover fingers or toes. By keeping these parts uncovered, you will be able to see if the bandage is too tight (Fig. 7-13, D). If fingers or toes become cold or begin to turn pale, blue or ashen, the bandage is too tight and should be loosened slightly.
- Apply additional dressings and

A STITCH IN TIME

It can be difficult to judge when a wound should receive stitches from a doctor. One rule of thumb is that stitches are needed when edges of skin do not fall together, the laceration involves the face or when any wound is over ½ inch long.

Stitches speed the healing process, lessen the chances of infection and improve the appearance of scars. They should be placed within the first few hours after the injury. The following major injuries often require stitches:

- Bleeding from an artery or uncontrolled bleeding.
- Wounds that show muscle or bone, involve joints, gape widely or involve hands or feet.
- Wounds from large or deeply embedded objects.
- Wounds from human or animal bites.
- Wounds that, if left unattended, could leave conspicuous scars, such as those on the face.

If you are caring for a wound and think that it may need stitches, it probably does. Once applied, stitches are easily cared for by gently applying a triple-antibiotic ointment to the skin around them, once or twice daily. If the wound gets red or swollen or if pus begins to form, a health-care provider should be notified.

Stitches in the face are often removed in less than a week. In joints, they are often removed after 2 weeks. Stitches on most other body parts require removal in 6 to 10 days. Some stitches dissolve naturally and do not require removal.

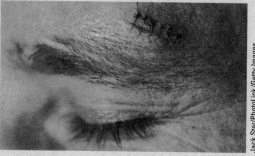

Jack Star/PhotoLink/Getty Images

FIGURE 7-13, A-D To apply a roller bandage, A, start by securing the bandage in place. B, Use overlapping turns to cover the dressing completely. C, Tie or tape the bandage in place. D, Check the fingers or toes for feeling, warmth and color.

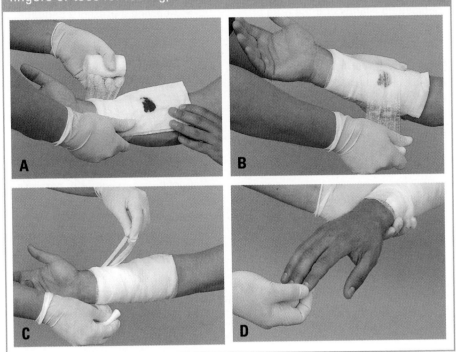

FIGURE 7-14 Elastic roller bandage.

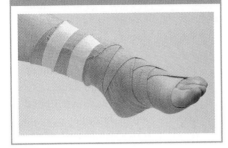

FIGURE 7-15, A-B A, To apply an elastic bandage, place the bandage against the skin and use overlapping turns. B, Gently stretch the bandage as you continue wrapping. The wrap should cover a long body section, like an arm or a calf, beginning at the point farthest from the heart.

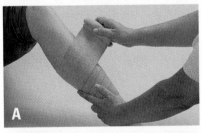

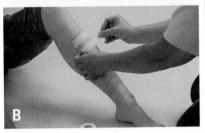

another bandage if blood soaks through the first bandage. Do not remove the blood-soaked bandages and dressings. Disturbing them may disrupt the formation of a clot and restart the bleeding.

Elastic Roller Bandages

Elastic roller bandages, sometimes called elastic wraps, are designed to keep continuous pressure on a body part. Elastic bandages are available in 2-, 3-, 4- and 6-inch widths. As with roller bandages, the first step in using an elastic bandage is to select the correct size of bandage. A narrow bandage would be used to wrap a hand or wrist. A medium-width bandage would be used for an arm or ankle. A wide bandage would be used to wrap a leg.

When properly applied, an elastic bandage may control swelling or support an injured limb, as in the care for an elapid (coral) snakebite (Fig. 7-14). (See Chapter 10 for more information on snake bites.) However, an improperly applied elastic bandage can restrict blood flow, which is not only painful but can also cause tissue damage if not corrected.

To apply an elastic roller bandage—
- Check the circulation of the limb beyond where you will be placing the bandage by checking for feeling, warmth and color.
- Place the end of the bandage against the skin and use overlapping turns (Fig. 7-15, A).
- Gently stretch the bandage as you continue wrapping (Fig. 7-15, B). The wrap should cover a long body section, like an arm or a calf, beginning at the point farthest from the heart. For a joint like a knee or ankle, use figure-eight turns to support the joint.

- Always check the area above and below the injury site for feeling, warmth and color, especially fingers and toes, after you have applied an elastic roller bandage. By checking both before and after bandaging, you will be able to tell if any tingling or numbness is from the bandaging or the injury.

Minor Open Wounds. In minor open wounds, such as abrasions, there is only a small amount of damage and bleeding.

To care for a minor open wound, follow these general guidelines:

- Use a barrier between your hand and the wound. If readily available, put on disposable gloves and place a sterile dressing on the wound.
- Apply direct pressure for a few minutes to control any bleeding.
- Wash the wound thoroughly with soap and water. If possible, irrigate an abrasion for 5 minutes with clean, running tap water.
- Apply triple-antibiotic ointment or cream to a minor wound if the person has no known allergies or sensitivities to the medication.
- Cover the wound with a sterile dressing and a bandage (or with an adhesive bandage) if it is still bleeding slightly or if the area of the wound is likely to come into contact with dirt or germs.

Major Open Wounds. A major open wound has serious tissue damage and severe bleeding. To care for a major open wound, you must act at once. Do not waste time washing the wound. Instead, follow these steps:

- Call 9-1-1 or the local emergency number.
- Put on disposable gloves. If you think that blood might splatter, you may need to wear eye protection.
- Control bleeding by—
  - Covering the wound with a dressing and firmly pressing against the wound with a gloved hand.
  - Applying a pressure bandage over the dressing to maintain pressure on the wound and to hold the dressing in place. If blood soaks through the bandage, do not remove the blood-soaked bandages. Instead, add more dressings and bandages to help absorb the blood.

Continue to monitor the person's airway, breathing and circulation. Observe the person closely for signals that may indicate that the person's condition is worsening, such as faster

A CONTINUOUS JOURNEY

There are about 60,000 miles of blood vessels in your body. These vessels act as a road map, directing blood to all parts of the body. As long as your heart beats, blood will flow through a continuous circuit of blood vessels known as arteries, veins and capillaries.

These blood vessels vary in diameter. The larger the vessel, the more blood that can flow through it. During rest, the heart pumps about 5.3 quarts of blood per minute through the blood vessels. During exercise, the blood vessels handle as much as six times this amount. This requires the blood vessels to be able to expand.

Arteries are large blood vessels that carry blood from the heart to all parts of the body. Because the blood in the arteries is closer to the pumping action of the heart, blood in the arteries travels faster and under greater pressure than blood in capillaries and veins. Blood flow in the arteries pulses with the heartbeat. Therefore, bleeding from the arteries is very fast and heavy. Arterial blood is usually bright red and, because it is under pressure, it spurts from the wound. This is one easily recognizable signal of severe bleeding.

Veins return blood from the body to the heart. Bleeding from the veins is slower, steadier and easier to control than arterial bleeding. Veins are damaged more often because they are closer to the skin's surface. Venous blood is dark red.

Capillaries are tiny blood vessels near the skin. They transfer oxygen and other nutrients to the body's cells. Bleeding from capillaries is usually slow and clots easily. Bleeding from scrapes and shallow cuts is from capillaries.

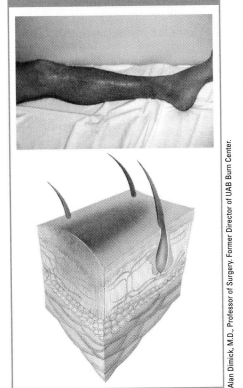

FIGURE 7-16 First-degree burn.

Alan Dimick, M.D., Professor of Surgery, Former Director of UAB Burn Center.

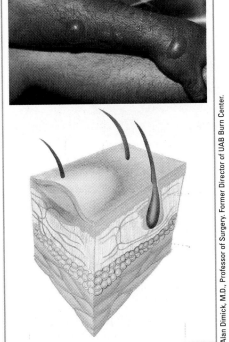

FIGURE 7-17 Second-degree burn.

Alan Dimick, M.D., Professor of Surgery, Former Director of UAB Burn Center.

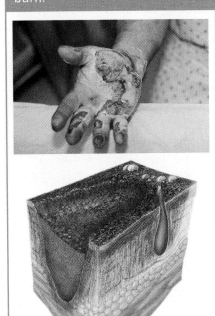

FIGURE 7-18 Third-degree burn.

Alan Dimick, M.D., Professor of Surgery, Former Director of UAB Burn Center.

or slower breathing, changes in skin color and restlessness.

- Keep the person from getting chilled or overheated.
- Have the person rest comfortably and reassure him or her.
- Wash your hands immediately after giving care.

BURNS

Burns are a special kind of soft tissue injury. Like other types of soft tissue injury, burns can damage the top layer of skin or the skin and the layers of fat, muscle and bone beneath.

Burns are classified by their sources: heat, chemicals, electricity and radiation (which includes burns caused by the sun). Burns also are classified by their depth. The deeper the burn, the more severe it is. The three levels of burns are: superficial (first degree) (Fig. 7-16), partial thick-

ness (second degree) (Fig. 7-17) and full thickness (third degree) (Fig. 7-18).

Critical Burns

A critical burn requires medical attention. These burns are potentially life threatening, disfiguring and disabling (Fig. 7-19). Unfortunately, it is often difficult to tell if a burn is critical. Even superficial burns can be critical if they affect a large area or certain body parts. You cannot judge a burn's severity by the pain that the burned person feels because nerve endings may be destroyed. You should always call 9-1-1 or the local emergency number if the burned person—

- Has trouble breathing.
- Has burns covering more than one body part or a large surface area.
- Has suspected burns to the airway. Burns to the mouth and nose may be a sign of this.

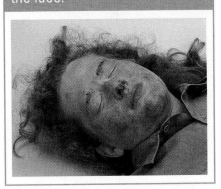

FIGURE 7-19 Critical burn to the face.

- Has burns to the head, neck, hands, feet or genitals.
- Has a full-thickness burn and is younger than age 5 or older than age 60.
- Has a burn resulting from chemicals, explosions or electricity.

HEAT   ELECTRIC
CHEMICAL   RADIATION

FIGURE 7-20, A-B A, Cool a thermal burn with large amounts of cold running water until pain is relieved. B, Cover a thermal burn loosely with a sterile dressing.

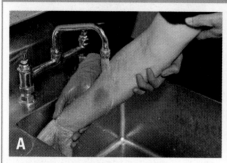
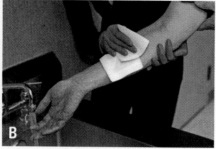

Caring for Burns

Follow these basic steps when caring for a thermal (heat) burn:

- Check the scene for safety.
- Stop the burning by removing the person from the source of the burn.
- Check for life-threatening conditions.
- Cool the burn with large amounts of cold running water (Fig. 7-20, A).
- Cover the burn loosely with a sterile dressing (Fig. 7-20, B).
- Prevent infection.
- Take steps to minimize shock. Keep the person from getting chilled or overheated.
- Comfort and reassure the person.

DO NOT—

- Apply ice or ice water except on a small, superficial burn and then for no more than 10 minutes. Ice can cause the body to lose heat and further damages delicate tissues.
- Touch a burn with anything except a clean covering.
- Remove pieces of clothing that stick to the burned area.
- Try to clean a severe burn.
- Break blisters.
- Use any kind of ointment on a severe burn.

Chemical Burns. When caring for chemical burns it is important to remember that the chemical will continue to burn as long as it is on the skin. You must remove the chemical from the body as quickly as possible. To do so, follow these steps:

1. If the burn was caused by dry chemicals, brush off the chemicals using gloved hands before flushing with tap water (under pressure). Be careful not to get the chemical on yourself or the person.
2. Flush the burn with large amounts of cool running water. Continue flushing the burn for at least 20 minutes or until EMS personnel arrive.
3. If an eye is burned by a chemical, flush the affected eye with water until EMS personnel arrive. Tip the head so that the affected eye is lower than the unaffected eye as you flush (Fig. 7-21).
4. If possible, have the person remove contaminated clothes to prevent further contamination while you continue to flush the area.

Be aware that chemicals can be inhaled, potentially damaging the airway or lungs.

CRITICAL FACTS

CHARACTERISTICS OF BURNS

- Superficial (first degree)
  - Involves only the top layer of skin.
  - Skin is red and dry, usually painful and the area may swell.
  - Usually heals within a week without permanent scarring.

- Partial thickness (second degree)
  - Involves the top layers of skin.
  - Skin is red; usually painful; has blisters that may open and weep clear fluid, making the skin appear wet; may appear mottled; and often swells.
  - Usually heals in 3 to 4 weeks and may scar.

- Full thickness (third degree)
  - May destroy all layers of skin and some or all of the underlying structures—fat, muscles, bones and nerves.
  - The skin may be brown or black (charred) with the tissue underneath sometimes appearing white, and can either be extremely painful or relatively painless (if the burn destroys nerve endings).
  - Healing may require medical assistance; scarring is likely.

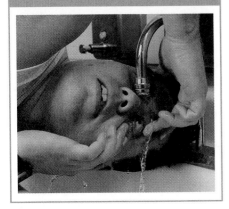

FIGURE 7-21 If an eye is burned by a chemical, flush the affected eye with water until EMS personnel arrive.

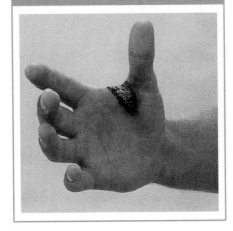

FIGURE 7-22 For an electrical burn, care for shock and thermal burns.

Electrical Burns. If you encounter an electrical burn, you should—

1. Never go near the person until you are sure he or she is not still in contact with the power source.
2. Call 9-1-1 in case of high-voltage electrocution, such as that caused by downed power lines.
3. Turn off the power at its source and care for any life-threatening conditions.
4. Be aware that electrocution can cause cardiac and respiratory emergencies. Therefore, be prepared to give cardiopulmonary resuscitation (CPR) or defibrillation.
5. Care for shock and thermal burns (Fig. 7-22).
6. Remember that anyone suffering from electric shock requires advanced medical care.

Radiation (Sun) Burns. Care for sunburn as you would for any other burn (Fig. 7-23). Always cool the burn and protect the area from further damage by keeping it out of the sun.

Preventing Burns

- Heat burns can be prevented by following safety practices that prevent fire and by being careful around sources of heat.
- Chemical burns can be prevented by following safety practices around all chemicals and by following manufacturers' guidelines when handling chemicals.
- Electrical burns can be prevented by following safety practices around electrical lines and equipment and by leaving outdoor areas when lightning could strike.

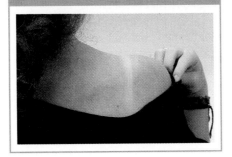

FIGURE 7-23 Care for sunburn as you would for any other burn.

- Sunburn can be prevented by wearing appropriate clothing and using sunscreen. Sunscreen should have a sun protection factor (SPF) of at least 15.

SPECIAL SITUATIONS

Severed Body Parts

If part of the body has been torn or cut off, call 9-1-1 or the local emergency number, then try to find the part and wrap it in sterile gauze or any clean material, such as a washcloth. Put the wrapped part in a plastic bag. Keep the part cold by placing the bag on ice, if possible, but do not freeze (Fig. 7-24). Be sure the part is taken to the hospital with the person. Doctors may be able to reattach it.

Embedded Objects

If an object, such as a knife or a piece of glass or metal, is embedded in a wound, do not remove it. Place several dressings around it to keep it from moving (Fig. 7-25, A). Bandage the dressings in place around the object (Fig. 7-25, B). If it is only a splinter in

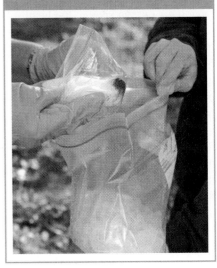

FIGURE 7-24 Wrap a severed body part in sterile gauze, put it in a plastic bag and put the bag on ice.

FIGURE 7-25, A-B A, Place several dressings around an embedded object to keep it from moving. B, Bandage the dressings in place around the object.

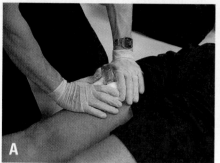
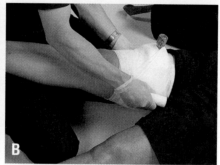

the surface of the skin, it can be removed with tweezers. After removing the splinter from the skin, wash the area with soap and water, rinsing the area with cold tap water for about 5 minutes. After drying the area, apply a triple antibiotic ointment or cream to the area and then cover it to keep it clean. If the splinter is in the eye, do not attempt to remove it. Call 9-1-1 or the local emergency number.

Nose Injuries

Nose injuries are usually caused by a blow from a blunt object. The result is often a nosebleed. High blood pressure or changes in altitude also can cause nosebleeds. In most cases, you can control bleeding by having the person sit with the head slightly forward while pinching the nostrils together for about 10 minutes (Fig. 7-26). Other methods of controlling bleeding include applying an ice pack (non-chemical) to the bridge of the nose or putting pressure on the upper lip just beneath the nose. Remember, ice should not be applied directly to the skin, as it can damage the skin tissue. Place a cloth between the ice and the skin. Seek medical attention if the bleeding persists or recurs or if the person says it results from high blood pressure.

FIGURE 7-26 To control a nosebleed, have the person lean forward and pinch the nostrils together until bleeding stops.

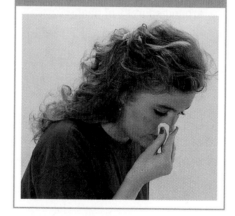

Mouth Injuries

With mouth injuries, you must make sure the person is able to breathe. Injuries to the mouth may cause breathing problems if blood or loose teeth obstruct the airway.

If the person is bleeding from the mouth and you do not suspect a serious head, neck or back injury, place the person in a seated position with the head tilted slightly forward. This will allow any blood to drain from the mouth. If this position is not possible, place the person on his or her side in

the recovery position to allow blood to drain from the mouth.

Lip Injuries

For injuries that penetrate the lip, place a rolled dressing between the lip and the gum. You can place another dressing on the outer surface of the lip. If the tongue is bleeding, apply a dressing and direct pressure. Applying cold to the lips or tongue can help reduce swelling and ease pain.

Tooth Injuries

If a person's tooth is knocked out, control the bleeding and save the tooth so it may possibly be reinserted. When the fibers and tissues are torn from the socket, it is important for the person to seek dental care within 30 minutes to an hour after the injury. Generally, the sooner the tooth is replaced, the better the chance is that it will survive.

If the person is conscious and able to cooperate, rinse out the mouth with cold tap water if available. You can control the bleeding by placing a rolled sterile dressing into the space left by the missing tooth (Fig. 7-27). Have the person gently bite down to

FIGURE 7-27 You can control the bleeding by placing a rolled sterile dressing and inserting it into the space left by the missing tooth.

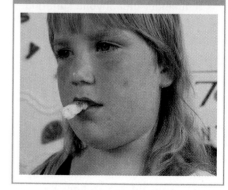

maintain pressure. To save the tooth, place it in milk if possible or cool water. Be careful to pick up the tooth by the crown (white part), rather than by the root.

Injuries to the Chest

The chest is the upper part of the trunk. The chest is shaped by 12 pairs of ribs. Ten of the pairs attach to the sternum (breastbone) in front and to the spine in back. Two pairs, the floating ribs, attach only to the spine. The rib cage, formed by the ribs, the sternum and the spine, protects vital organs, such as the heart, major blood vessels and the lungs. Also in the chest are the esophagus, trachea and muscles of respiration.

Chest injuries are a leading cause of trauma deaths each year. Injuries to the chest may result from a wide variety of causes, such as motor vehicle crashes, falls, sports mishaps and crushing or penetrating forces. Chest injuries may involve the bones that form the chest cavity or the organs or other structures in the cavity itself.

Chest wounds are either open or closed. Open chest wounds occur when an object, such as a knife or bullet, penetrates the chest wall. Fractured ribs may break through the skin to cause an open chest injury. A closed chest wound does not break the skin. Closed chest wounds are generally caused by blunt objects, such as steering wheels.

You may recognize some of the signals of a serious chest injury from previous discussions in this manual about respiratory distress, soft tissue injuries and musculoskeletal injuries. They include—

- Trouble breathing.
- Severe pain at the site of the injury.
- Flushed, pale, ashen or bluish skin.
- Obvious deformity, such as that caused by a fracture.

- Coughing up blood (may be bright red or dark like coffee grounds).
- Bruising at the site of a blunt injury, such as that caused by a seat belt.
- A "sucking" noise or distinct sound when the person breathes.

Rib Fractures. Rib fractures are usually caused by direct force to the chest. Although painful, a simple rib fracture is rarely life threatening (Fig. 7-28). A person with a fractured rib generally remains calm, but his or her breathing is shallow because normal or deep breathing is painful. The person will usually attempt to ease the pain by supporting the injured area with a hand or arm.

Rib fractures are less common in children because children's ribs are so flexible that they bend rather than break. However, the forces that can cause a rib fracture in adults can severely bruise the lung tissue of children, which can be a life-threatening injury. Look for signals, such as what caused the injury, bruising on the chest and trouble breathing, to determine if a child has potential chest injury.

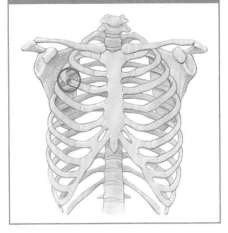

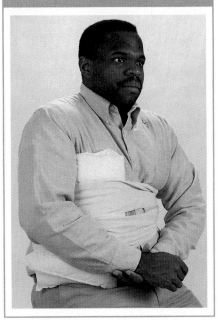

Care for Rib Fractures. If you suspect a fractured rib, have the person rest in a position that will make breathing easier. Do not move the person if you suspect a head, neck or back injury. Call 9-1-1 or the local emergency number. Binding the person's upper arm to the chest on the injured side will help support the injured area and make breathing more comfortable. You can use an object, such as a pillow or rolled blanket, to support and immobilize the area (Fig. 7-29). Monitor breathing and skin condition, and take steps to minimize shock.

Puncture Wounds to the Chest. Puncture wounds to the chest range from minor to life threatening. Stab and gunshot wounds are examples of puncture injuries. The penetrating object can injure any structure or organ within the chest, including the lungs. A puncture injury can allow air to enter the chest through the

FIGURE 7-30 If the injury penetrates the rib cage, air can pass freely in and out of the chest cavity, and the person cannot breathe normally.

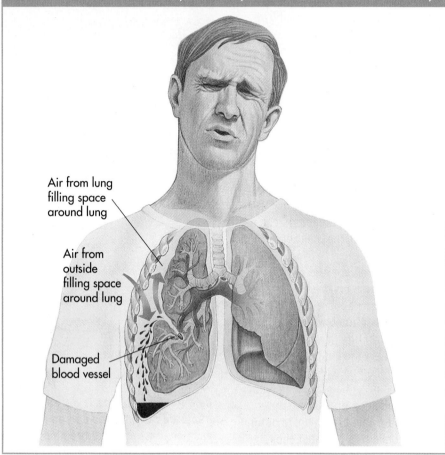

Air from lung filling space around lung

Air from outside filling space around lung

Damaged blood vessel

wound. Air in the chest cavity does not allow the lungs to function normally.

Puncture wounds cause varying degrees of internal and external bleeding. A puncture wound to the chest is a life-threatening injury. If the injury penetrates the rib cage, air can pass freely in and out of the chest cavity, and the person cannot breathe normally. With each breath the person takes, you will hear a sucking sound coming from the wound. This sound is the primary signal of a penetrating chest injury called a *sucking chest wound* (Fig. 7-30). Without proper care, the person's condition will worsen. The affected lung or lungs will fail to function, and breathing will become more difficult. Call 9-1-1 or the local emergency number.

Care for a Sucking Chest Wound. To care for a sucking chest wound, cover the wound with a large occlusive dressing (Fig. 7-31). A piece of plastic wrap or a plastic bag folded several times and placed over the wound makes an effective occlusive dressing.

FIGURE 7-31 An occlusive dressing keeps air from entering the wound when the person inhales, and having an open corner allows air to escape when the person exhales.

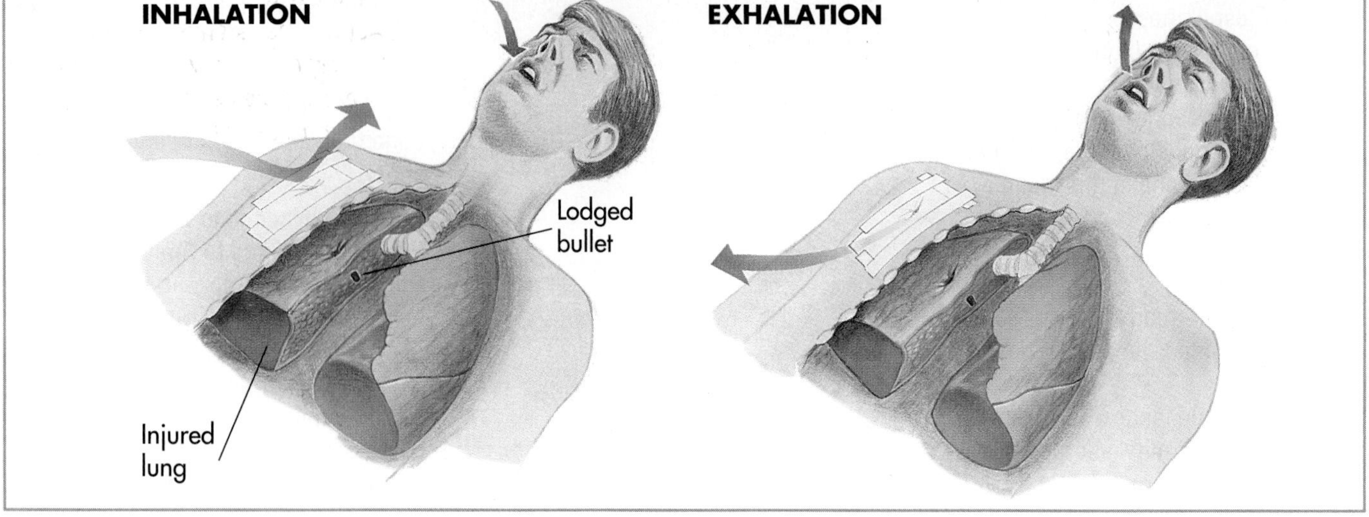

INHALATION

EXHALATION

Lodged bullet

Injured lung

Tape the dressing in place, except for one side or corner that should remain loose. A taped-down dressing keeps air from entering the wound when the person inhales, and having an open corner allows air to escape when the person exhales. If these materials are not available to use as dressings, use a folded cloth. Call 9-1-1 or the local emergency number. Take steps to minimize shock.

Abdominal Injury

Like a chest injury, an injury to the abdomen may be either open or closed. Injuries to the abdomen can be very painful. Even with a closed wound, the rupture of an organ can cause serious internal bleeding that results in shock. It is especially difficult to determine if a person has an internal abdominal injury if he or she is unconscious.

Always suspect an abdominal injury in a person who has multiple injuries. Signals of serious abdominal injury include—

- Severe pain.
- Bruising.
- External bleeding.
- Nausea.
- Vomiting (sometimes containing blood).
- Weakness.
- Thirst.
- Pain, tenderness or a tight feeling in the abdomen.
- Organs protruding from the abdomen.
- Rigid abdominal muscles.
- Other signals of shock.

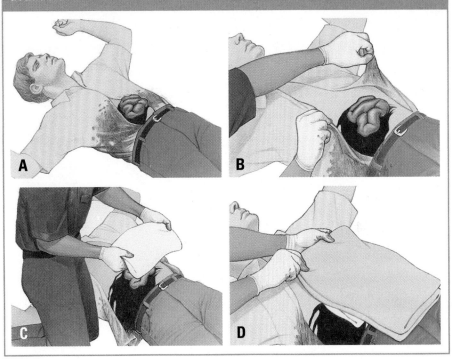

FIGURE 7-32, A-D A, Wounds that break through the abdomen can cause the organs to protrude. B, Carefully remove clothing from around the wound, C, cover the organs loosely with a moist, sterile dressing and D, cover the dressings loosely with plastic wrap, if available.

Care for Abdominal Injuries. With a severe open injury, abdominal organs sometimes protrude through the wound (Fig. 7-32, A). To care for an open wound to the abdomen, follow these steps:

1. Call 9-1-1 or the local emergency number.
2. Put on disposable gloves or use another barrier.
3. Carefully position the person on his or her back with the knees bent, if that position does not cause pain.
4. Do not apply direct pressure.
5. Do not push any protruding organs back in.
6. Remove clothing from around the wound (Fig. 7-32, B).
7. Apply moist, sterile dressings loosely over the wound. (Warm tap water can be used.) (Fig. 7-32, C.)
8. Cover dressings loosely with plastic wrap, if available (Fig. 7-32, D).

Controlling External Bleeding

(BLEEDING)

> *(**TIP:** Use disposable gloves and other personal protective equipment.)*

STEP 1
CHECK scene, then **CHECK** person.

STEP 2
Obtain consent.

STEP 3
Cover wound with a sterile dressing.

STEP 4
Apply direct pressure until bleeding stops.

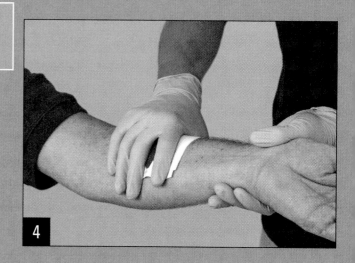

OBJECT -
PRESS DRESSINGS
AROUND OBJECT
ROLLER BANDAGE

STEP 5

Cover dressing with bandage. *+ SECURE END*

STEP 6

If bleeding does not stop—

- Apply additional dressings and bandages.
- Take steps to minimize shock.
- **CALL 9-1-1** if not already done.

*(**NOTE:** Wash hands with soap and water after giving care.)*

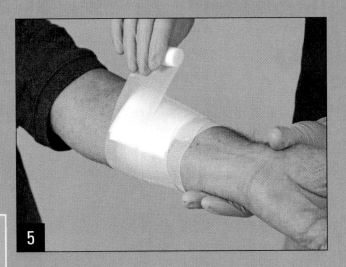

5

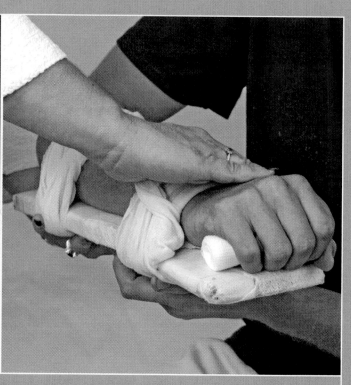

8

If you suspect a serious muscle, bone or joint injury, keep the injured part from moving.

Chapter 8

Injuries to Muscles, Bones and Joints

It's a beautiful, sunny Saturday afternoon, and where are you? In the hospital emergency room, that's where, with a knee hurting so bad you had to borrow crutches to get there. Maybe it's time to give up the weekend athletics. You pass the time waiting your turn and watching other visitors. They come in all ages and sizes. Here's a 14-year-old football player complete with anxious parents and a throbbing ankle. Watching TV is the 40-something would-be rock climber—who couldn't. An ambulance pulls up and an ashen, gray-haired man with both legs in splints is wheeled by the waiting room. What do all of these people have in common? They've each got some sort of injury to a muscle, bone or joint.

Injuries to muscles, bones and joints happen often. They happen to people of all ages at home, work and play. They are painful and they make life difficult. A person may fall and bruise the muscles of one leg, making walking painful. Equipment may fall on a worker and break bones. A person bracing one hand against the dashboard in a car accident may injure the bones at the shoulder and disable the arm. A skier may fall and twist a leg, tearing muscles and making it impossible to stand or move.

While painful, these injuries are rarely life threatening. If they are not recognized and cared for, however, they can cause serious problems, even disability.

MUSCLES

The body's skeleton is made up of bones, muscles and the tendons and ligaments that connect them. Together, they give the body shape and stability. Bones and muscles connect to form various parts of the body. They work together to allow the body to move.

Muscles are soft tissues. The body has over 600 muscles, most of which are attached to bones by strong tissues called *tendons* (Fig. 8-1). Unlike other soft tissues, muscles are able to shorten and lengthen—contract and relax. This contracting and relaxing is what makes the body move (Fig. 8-2). The brain directs the muscles to move through the spinal cord, a pathway of nerves in the spine. Tiny jolts of electricity called *electrical impulses* travel through the nerves to the muscles.

They cause the muscles to contract. When the muscles contract, they pull at the bones, causing motion at a joint.

Injuries to the brain, the spinal cord or the nerves can affect muscle control. When nerves lose control of muscles, it is called *paralysis*. When a muscle is injured, a nearby muscle often takes over for the injured one.

FIGURE 8-1 The body has over 600 muscles, most of which are attached to bones by strong tissues called *tendons*.

FRONT VIEW

- Face muscles
- Neck muscles
- Deltoid
- Biceps
- Extensors of wrist and fingers
- Quadriceps muscles
- Extensors of foot and toes
- Chest muscles
- Abdominal muscles
- Groin muscles

BACK VIEW

- Neck muscles
- Back muscles
- Gluteus maximus
- Hamstring muscles
- Calf muscles
- Achilles tendon
- Deltoid
- Triceps
- Extensors of wrist and fingers

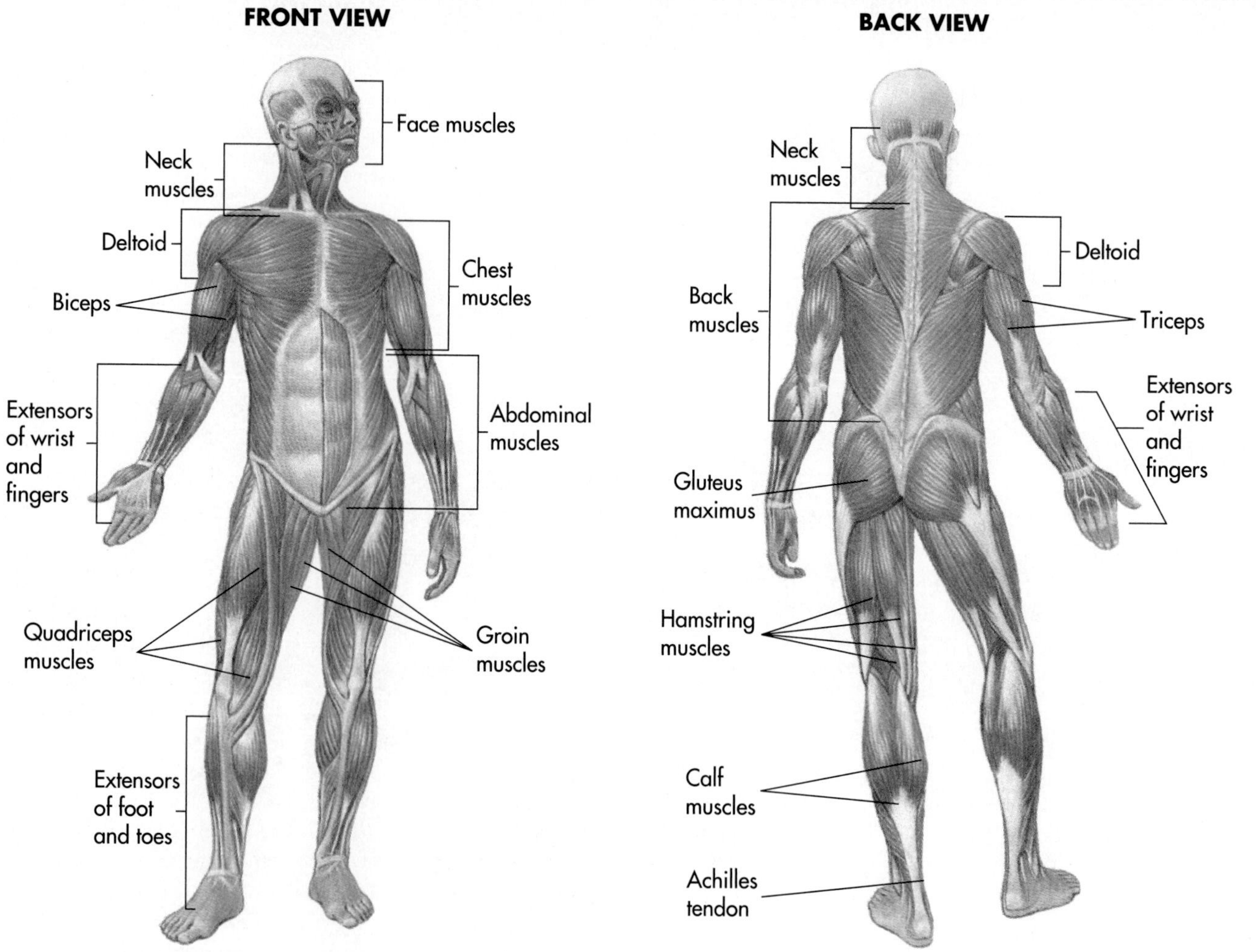

REST
Immobilization
Cold
Elevation

Contract
Relax

Contract
Relax

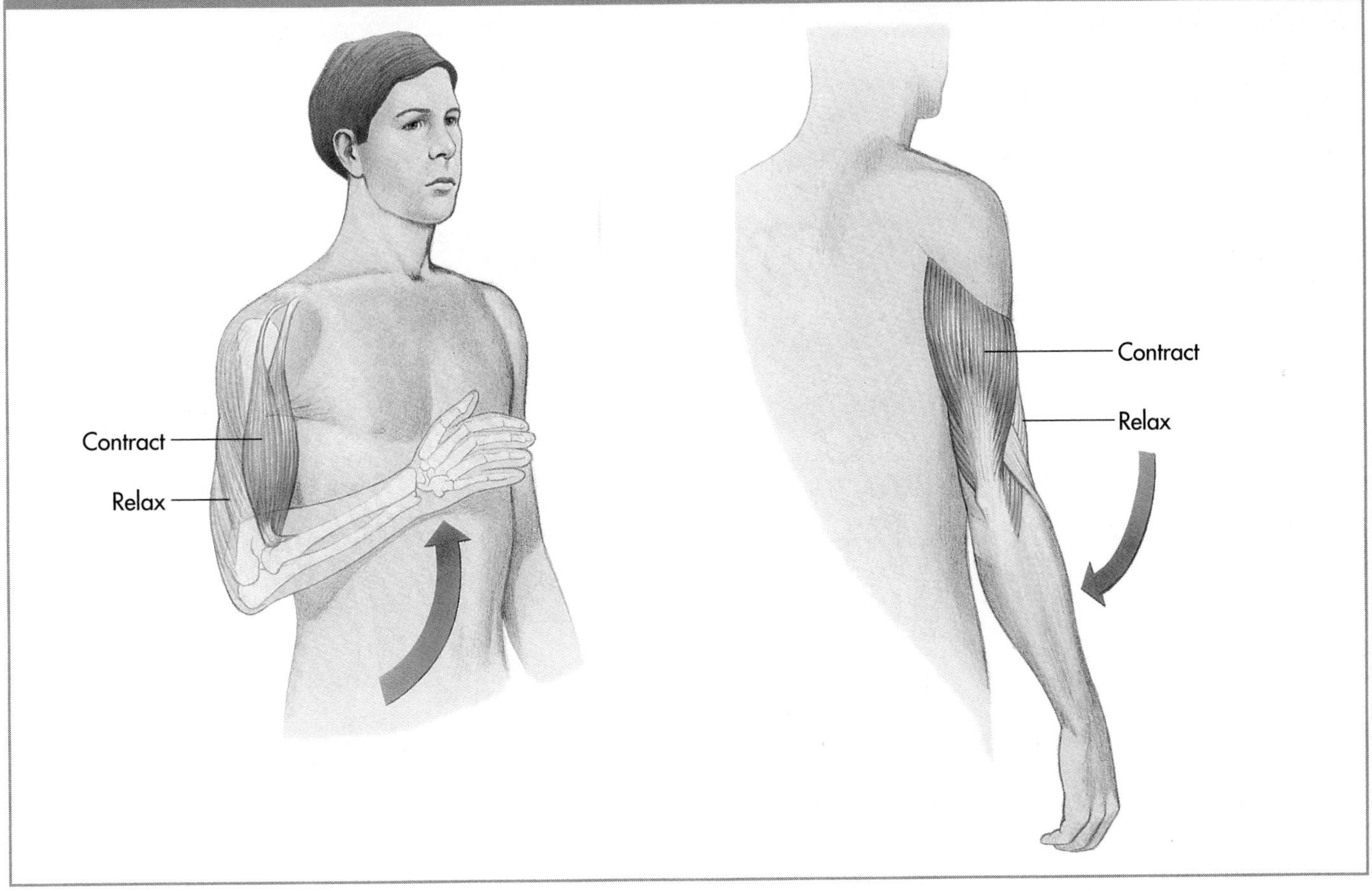

BONES

Approximately 200 bones in various sizes and shapes form the skeleton (Fig. 8-3). The skeleton protects many of the organs inside the body. Bones are hard and dense. Because they are strong and rigid, they are not injured easily. Bones have a rich supply of blood and nerves. Bone injuries can bleed and they usually hurt. If the injury is not cared for, the bleeding can become life threatening. Bones weaken with age. Children have more flexible bones than adults; their bones break less easily. If a child sustains a fracture to the growth plate, however,

it can affect future bone growth. Older adults have more brittle bones. Sometimes they break surprisingly easily. This gradual weakening of bones is called *osteoporosis*.

JOINTS

The ends of two or more bones coming together at one place form a joint (Fig. 8-4). Strong, tough bands called *ligaments* hold the bones at a joint together. All joints have a normal range of movement—an area in which they can move freely without too much stress or strain. When joints are

forced beyond this range, ligaments stretch and tear.

TYPES OF INJURIES

The four basic types of injuries to muscles, bones and joints are fractures, dislocations, strains and sprains. They happen in a variety of ways.

Fractures

A fracture is a complete break, a chip or a crack in a bone (Fig. 8-5). A fall, a blow or sometimes even a twisting movement can cause a fracture. Fractures are open or closed. An open fracture involves an open wound. It

FIGURE 8-3 Approximately 200 bones in various sizes and shapes form the skeleton. The skeleton protects many of the organs inside the body.

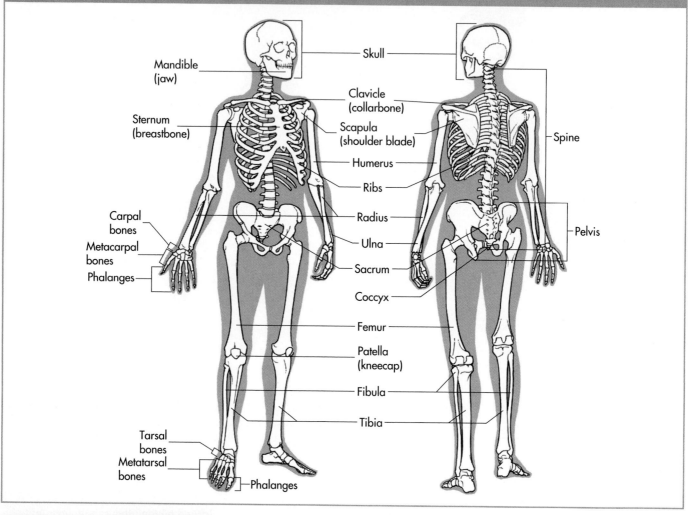

Mandible (jaw) • Skull • Clavicle (collarbone) • Sternum (breastbone) • Scapula (shoulder blade) • Spine • Humerus • Ribs • Carpal bones • Radius • Metacarpal bones • Ulna • Pelvis • Phalanges • Sacrum • Coccyx • Femur • Patella (kneecap) • Fibula • Tibia • Tarsal bones • Metatarsal bones • Phalanges

FIGURE 8-4 The ends of two or more bones coming together at one place form a joint.

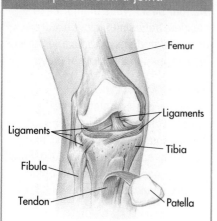

Femur • Ligaments • Ligaments • Tibia • Fibula • Tendon • Patella

occurs when bone ends tear through the skin. An object that goes into the skin and breaks the bone, such as a bullet, also can cause an open fracture. In a closed fracture the skin is not broken.

Closed fractures are more common, but open fractures are more dangerous because they carry a risk of infection and severe bleeding. In general, fractures are life threatening only if they involve breaks in large bones such as the thigh, sever an artery or affect breathing. Since you cannot always tell if a person has a fracture,

you should consider the cause of the injury. A fall from a height or a motor vehicle crash could signal a possible fracture.

Dislocations

Dislocations are usually more obvious than fractures. A dislocation is the movement of a bone at a joint away from its normal position (Fig. 8-6). This movement is usually caused by a violent force tearing the ligaments that hold the bones in place. When a bone is moved out of place, the joint no longer functions. The displaced bone

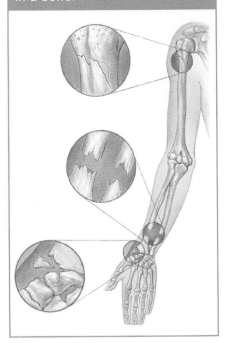

FIGURE 8-5 A fracture is a complete break, chip or crack in a bone.

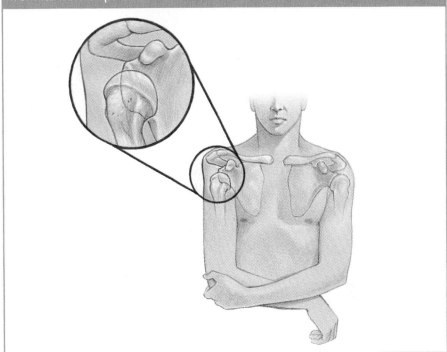

FIGURE 8-6 A dislocation is the movement of a bone at a joint away from its normal position.

end often forms a bump, a ridge or a hollow that does not normally exist.

Sprains

A sprain is the tearing of ligaments at a joint (Fig. 8-7, A). Mild sprains may swell but usually heal quickly. The person might not feel much pain and is active again soon. If a person ignores the signals of swelling and pain and becomes active too soon, the joint will not heal properly and will remain weak. There is a good chance it will become reinjured, only this time more severely. A severe sprain can also involve a fracture or dislocation of the bones at the joint. The joints most easily injured are at the ankle, knee, wrist and fingers.

Strains

A strain is a stretching and tearing of muscles or tendons (Fig. 8-7, B). Strains are often caused by lifting

SIGNALS OF SERIOUS MUSCLE, BONE OR JOINT INJURIES

Always suspect a serious injury when any of the following signals are present:

- Significant deformity

- Bruising and swelling

- Inability to use the affected part normally

- Bone fragments sticking out of a wound

- Person feels bones grating; person felt or heard a snap or pop at the time of injury

- The injured area is cold and numb

- Cause of the injury suggests that the injury may be severe

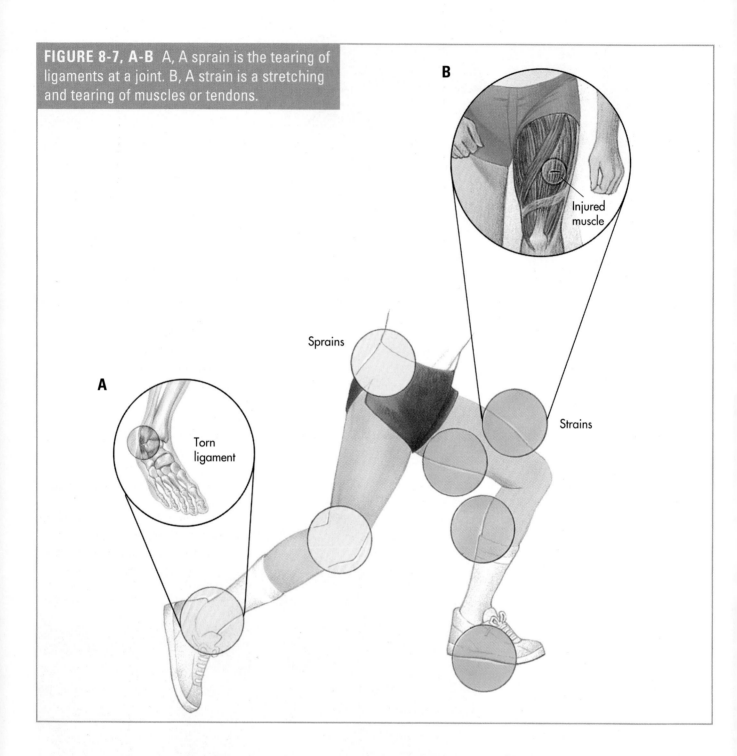

FIGURE 8-7, A-B A, A sprain is the tearing of ligaments at a joint. B, A strain is a stretching and tearing of muscles or tendons.

A Torn ligament

B Injured muscle

Sprains

Strains

something heavy or working a muscle too hard. They usually involve the muscles in the neck, back, thigh or the back of the lower leg. Some strains can reoccur, especially in the neck and back.

How can you tell how bad the injury is to a muscle, bone or joint? Often you cannot. Sometimes an X-ray, computer aided tomography (CAT scan) or magnetic resonance imaging (MRI) is needed to determine the extent of the injury.

Signals of Severe Injury

Certain signals can indicate that the injury may be severe. One of the most common signals is pain. The injured area may be painful to touch and move. The area may be swollen and red or bruised. The area may be twisted or

FIGURE 8-8 A severely injured bone or joint may appear deformed.

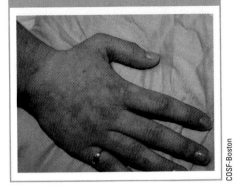

COSF-Boston

CRITICAL FACTS

SPLINTING

- Splint only if the person must be moved or transported by someone other than emergency medical personnel.
- Splint only if you can do so without causing more pain.
- Splint an injury in the position you find it.
- Splint the injured area and the bones or joints above and below the injury.
- Check for circulation (feeling, warmth and color) before and after splinting.

strangely bent (Fig. 8-8). It may have abnormal lumps, ridges and hollows.

A good way to tell if an area is not normal is to compare it with an uninjured part. For example, if you compare an arm you think may be fractured or dislocated with the uninjured one, you may be able to spot something that looks strange or out of place. The person may hear a snap or pop at the time of the injury or feel bones grating. Hands and fingers or feet and toes may feel numb or tingly.

Caring for Muscle, Bone or Joint Injuries

The general care for injuries to muscles, bone and joints includes following **RICE**:

Rest—Do not move or straighten the injured area.

Immobilize—Stabilize the injured area in the position it was found. Splint the injured part ONLY if the person must be moved and it does not cause more pain.

Cold—Fill a plastic bag or wrap ice with a damp cloth and apply ice to the injured area for periods of 20 minutes. If continued icing is needed, remove the pack for 20 minutes, and then replace it. Place a thin barrier between the ice and bare skin (Fig. 8-9).

Elevate—**Do not** elevate the injured part if it causes more pain.

Splinting Injuries. Splinting is a method of immobilizing an injured part and should ONLY be used if you have to move or transport the person to seek medical attention and if it does not cause more pain. Splint an injury in the position in which you find it. For fractures, splint the joint above and joint below the point of injury. For sprains, splint the bone above and bone below the point of the injury. If you are not sure if the injury is a fracture or a sprain, splint both the bones and joints above and below the point

of injury. Check for circulation (feeling, warmth and color) before and after splinting to make sure the splint is not too tight.

There are many methods of splinting, including—

- **Anatomic splints.** The person's body is the splint. For example, you can splint an arm to the chest or an injured leg to the uninjured leg (Fig. 8-10).
- **Soft splints.** Soft materials such as a folded blanket, towel, pillow or folded triangular bandage can be splint materials (Fig. 8-11). A sling is a specific kind of soft splint that uses a triangular bandage tied to

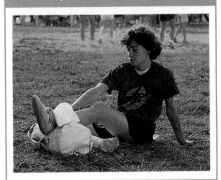

FIGURE 8-9 Applying ice can help control swelling and reduce pain.

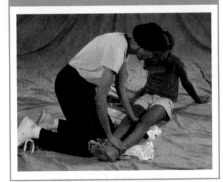

FIGURE 8-10 An anatomic splint uses a part of the body as the splint.

FIGURE 8-11 Folded blankets, towels, pillows and a triangular bandage tied as a sling can be used as soft splints.

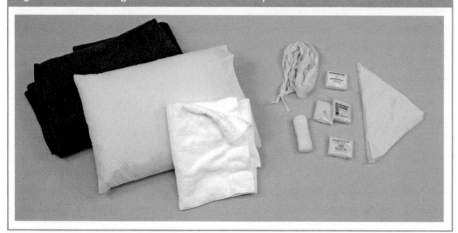

support an injured arm, wrist or hand.

- **Rigid splints.** Boards, folded magazines or newspapers, or metal strips that do not have any sharp edges, can serve as splints (Fig. 8-12).
- **The ground.** An injured leg stretched out on the ground is splinted by the ground.

After you have splinted the injury, apply ice to the injured area. Keep the person from getting chilled or overheated and be reassuring.

Some injuries, such as a broken finger, do not require you to call 9-1-1 or the local emergency number but still need medical attention. When transporting the person, have someone else drive, if possible, so you can keep an eye on the person and give necessary care. Injuries to the hip or thigh are rarely life threatening, but might require an ambulance to transport the injured person without bending at the hip.

FIGURE 8-12 Boards, folded newspapers and magazines can be used as rigid splints.

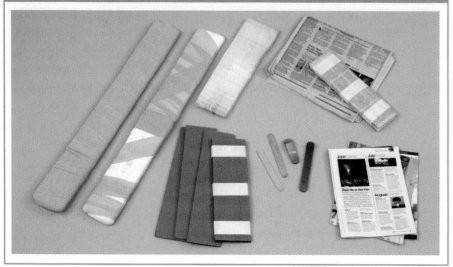

Head, Neck and Back Injuries

Although head, neck and back injuries make up only a small fraction of all injuries, these injuries may cause unintentional death or lifelong neurological damage. Each year, approximately 11,000 Americans suffer a head, neck or back injury. Most of them are males under 40 years of age. Motor vehicle crashes cause about half of these injuries. Falls, sports accidents and acts of violence cause the rest.

Injuries to the head, neck or back can cause paralysis, speech or memory problems or other disabling conditions. These injuries can damage bone and soft tissue, including the brain and spinal cord. Since generally only X-rays, CAT scans or MRIs can show the severity of a head, neck or back injury, you should always care for such injuries as if they were serious.

An injury to the brain can cause bleeding inside the skull (Fig. 8-13).

FIGURE 8-13 Injuries to the head can rupture blood vessels in the brain. Pressure builds within the skull as blood accumulates, causing brain injury.

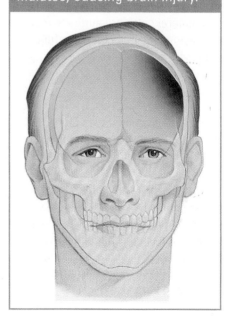

A

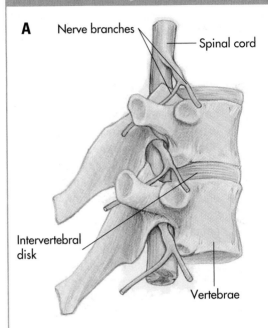

Nerve branches
Spinal cord
Intervertebral disk
Vertebrae

B

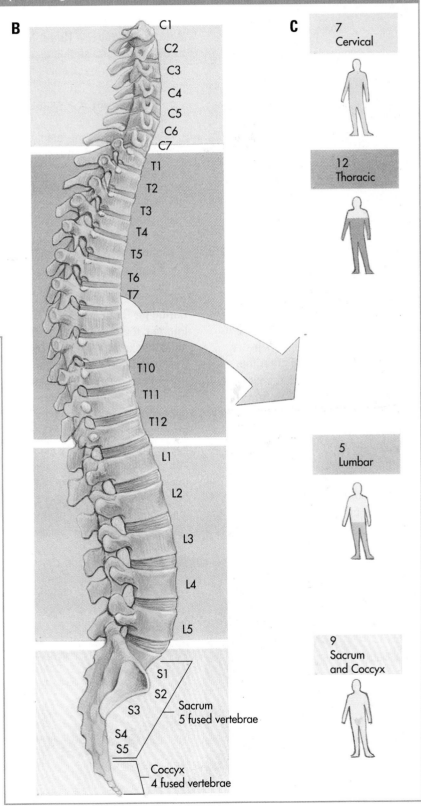

C1
C2
C3
C4
C5
C6
C7
T1
T2
T3
T4
T5
T6
T7
T10
T11
T12
L1
L2
L3
L4
L5
S1
S2
S3
Sacrum 5 fused vertebrae
S4
S5
Coccyx 4 fused vertebrae

C

7 Cervical

12 Thoracic

5 Lumbar

9 Sacrum and Coccyx

The blood can build up and cause pressure, resulting in more damage. The first and most important signal of brain injury is a change in the level of the person's consciousness. He or she may be dizzy or confused or may become unconscious.

The spine is a strong, flexible column of small bones that support the head and trunk (Fig. 8-14, A-C). The spinal cord runs through the circular openings of the small bones called the *vertebrae*. The vertebrae are separated from each other by cushions of cartilage called *disks*. Nerves originating in the brain form branches extending to various parts of the body through openings in the vertebrae. Injuries to the back can fracture vertebrae and tear ligaments. In some cases the vertebrae can shift and cut or squeeze the spinal cord. This can paralyze and even kill the person.

COMMON CAUSES OF BACK INJURY

Motor Vehicle Crashes	47.5%
Falls	22.9%
Acts of Violence	13.8%
Sports Injuries	8.9%
Other	6.8%

Source: National Spinal Cord Injury Information Network, 2005.

Signals of Head, Neck and Back Injuries. When you are dealing with an injured person, try to determine if there is a head, neck or back injury involved. Think about whether the forces involved were great enough to cause one of these injuries. Someone may have fallen from a height or struck his or her head diving. He or she might have been in a motor vehicle crash and had not been wearing a safety belt. Maybe the person was thrown from the vehicle. Perhaps the person was struck by lightning or maybe a bullet that struck the spine pierced his

or her back. Always suspect a head, neck or back injury if a person is unconscious and/or if his or her safety helmet is broken.

When to Suspect a Head, Neck or Back Injury. You should also suspect a head, neck or back injury if the person—

- Was involved in a motor vehicle crash.
- Was injured as a result of a fall from greater than a standing height.
- Complains of neck or back pain.
- Has tingling or weakness in the extremities.
- Is not fully alert.
- Appears to be intoxicated.
- Appears to be frail or over 65 years of age.

Caring for Head, Neck and Back Injuries. If you think a person has a head, neck or back injury, call 9-1-1 or the local emergency number. While you are waiting for emergency medical services (EMS) personnel to arrive, the best care you can give is to minimize movement of the person's head and spine. Do this by placing your hands on both sides of the person's head. Gently hold the person's head in line with the body, in the position in which you found it and support it in that position until EMS personnel arrive (Fig. 8-15, A-B). If

the head is sharply turned to one side, DO NOT move it. Support it in the position found (Fig. 8-15, C).

If a person with a suspected head, neck or back injury is wearing a helmet, do not remove it unless necessary to assess the person's airway and you are specifically trained to do so. Minimize movement using the same technique you would use if the person were not wearing headgear.

The person may become confused, drowsy or unconscious. Breathing may stop. The person may be bleeding. If the person is unconscious, you need to keep the airway open and check breathing, as you learned in Chapter 4. You should control severe bleeding and keep the person from getting chilled or overheated, as you learned in Chapter 2. Remember, if you think the person may have a head, neck or back injury, call 9-1-1 or the local emergency number.

Chest Injuries

Injuries to the chest may be caused by falls, sports mishaps and crushing or penetrating forces. Chest injuries range from a simple broken rib to serious life-threatening injuries. Although painful, a simple broken rib is rarely life threatening.

A person with a broken rib will take small, shallow breaths because

FIGURE 8-15, A-C Gently hold the person's head in line with the body, in the position in which you found it, and support it in that position until EMS personnel arrive.

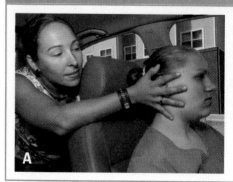
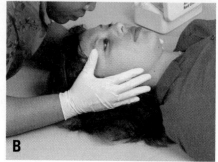
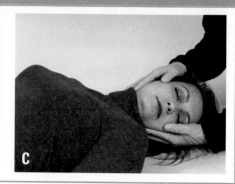

normal or deep breathing is painful. The person will experience discomfort or pain at the site of the injury and will usually try to ease the pain by supporting the area with a hand or arm. If the injury is serious, the person will have trouble breathing. The person's skin may appear flushed, pale or ashen and he or she may cough up blood. Remember that a person with a serious chest injury may also have a back injury.

If you suspect injured ribs, have the person rest in a position that will make breathing easier. Binding the person's arm to the chest on the injured side will help support the injured area and make breathing more comfortable. You can use an object, such as a pillow or folded blanket, to support and immobilize the area. If you think the injury is serious or the spine has also been injured, do not move the person. If the person is standing, do not lie the person down. Continue to watch the person until EMS personnel arrive and take over.

Pelvic Injuries

The large, heavy bones of the hip are called the *pelvis*. Like the chest, injury to the pelvic bones can range from simple to life threatening. Because these large bones help protect important organs inside the body, severe forces can cause heavy internal bleeding. Although a serious injury may be immediately obvious, some may develop over time.

Because an injury to the pelvis can also injure the lower spine, it is best not to move the person. If possible, try to keep the person lying flat. Watch for signals of internal bleeding and take steps to minimize shock until EMS personnel arrive.

THE BREAKING POINT

Osteoporosis is a bone disease that people usually have for decades before they experience signals. People do not usually become aware they have this "silent" disease until after the age of 60.

28 million Americans have osteoporosis and 80 percent of those affected are women. Fair-skinned women with ancestors from northern Europe, the British Isles, Japan or China are most likely to develop osteoporosis. One-and-a-half million spine, hip, wrist and other fractures occur annually in the United States because of osteoporosis. An American woman's risk of hip fracture alone is equal to her combined risk of breast, uterine and ovarian cancer.

Osteoporosis occurs when the calcium content of bone decreases. Normal bones are hard, dense tissues that endure great stresses. Calcium is a key to bone growth, development and repair. When the calcium content of bones decreases, bones become frail and less dense. They are less able to repair the normal damage they incur. This leaves bones, especially hip, back and wrist, more prone to fractures. These fractures may occur with only a little force. Some even occur without force. The person may be taking a walk or washing dishes when the fracture occurs.

Osteoporosis can begin as early as age 30. The amount of calcium a person absorbs from his or her diet declines with age, making calcium intake more important as a person gets older.

Building strong bones before age 35 is the key to preventing osteoporosis. Calcium and exercise are necessary to bone building. Three to four daily servings of low-fat dairy products should provide enough calcium. Vitamin D also is necessary because it helps the body to absorb calcium to form strong bones. Exposure to sunshine enables the body to make vitamin D. People who do not receive adequate exposure to the sun need to eat foods that contain vitamin D. The best sources are vitamin-fortified milk and fatty fish, such as tuna, salmon and eel. Exposure to the sun should not, however, cause a burn or deep tan, both of which increase the risk of skin cancer.

People who do not take in adequate calcium may be able to make up for the loss by taking calcium supplements. Some are combined with vitamin D. Before taking a calcium supplement, however, consult your health-care provider. Many highly advertised calcium supplements are ineffective because they do not dissolve in the body.

Weight-bearing exercise increases bone density and the activity of bone-building cells. Regular exercise may reduce the rate of bone loss by promoting new bone formation. It may also stimulate the skeletal system to repair itself. An effective exercise program, such as aerobics, jogging or walking, involves the weight-bearing bones and muscles of the legs.

If you have questions about your health and osteoporosis, consult your health-care provider.

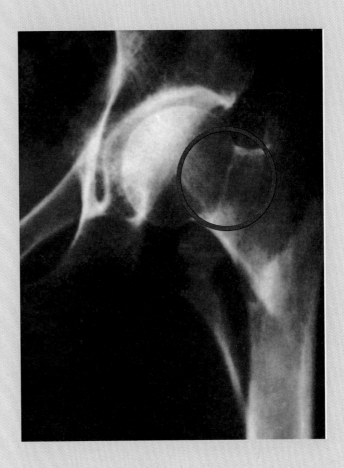

Applying an Anatomic Splint

CHECK the scene for safety. **CHECK** the injured person following standard precautions. **CALL** 9-1-1 or the local emergency number if necessary. To **CARE** for a person who has an injured limb—

STEP 1
Obtain consent.

STEP 2
Support the injured body part above and below the site of the injury.

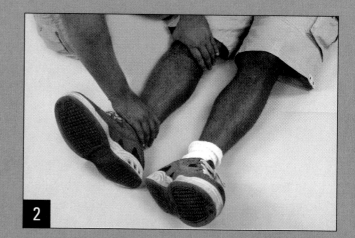

STEP 3
Check for feeling, warmth and color.

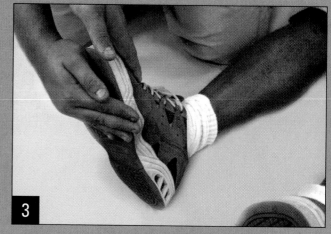

STEP 4
Place several folded triangular bandages above and below the injured body part.

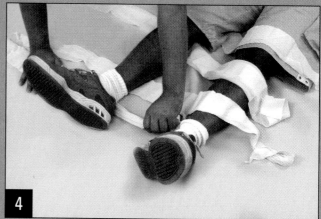

STEP 5

Place the uninjured body part next to the injured body part.

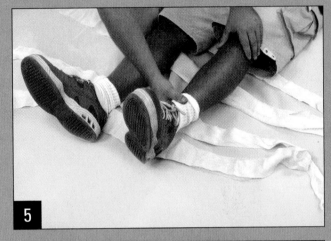

STEP 6

Tie triangular bandages securely.

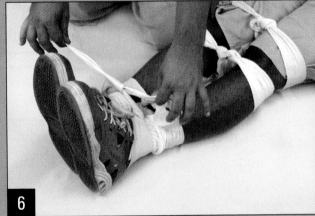

STEP 7

Recheck for feeling, warmth and color.

(*TIP: If you are not able to check warmth and color because a sock or shoe is in place, check for feeling.*)

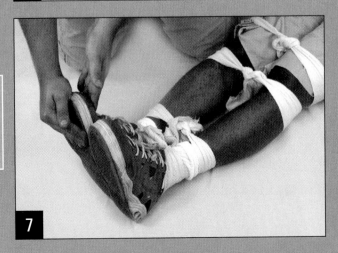

Applying a Soft Splint

CHECK the scene for safety. CHECK the injured person following standard precautions. CALL 9-1-1 or the local emergency number if necessary. To CARE for a person who has an injured limb—

STEP 1
Obtain consent.

STEP 2
Support the injured body part above and below the site of the injury.

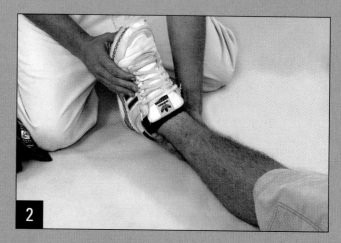

STEP 3
Check for feeling, warmth and color.

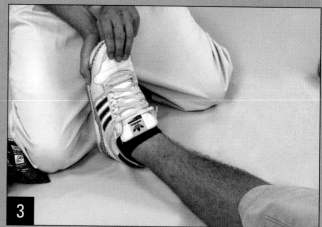

STEP 4
Place several folded triangular bandages above and below the injured body part.

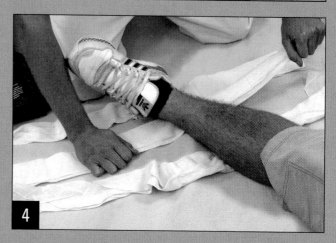

STEP 5

Gently wrap a soft object (a folded blanket or pillow) around the injured body part.

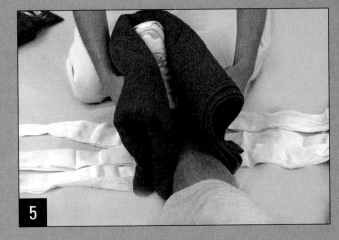

STEP 6

Tie triangular bandages securely with knots.

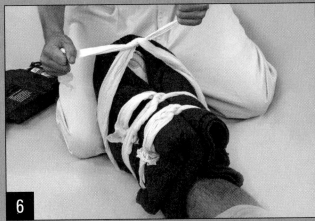

STEP 7

Recheck for feeling, warmth and color.

(**TIP:** *If you are not able to check warmth and color because a sock or shoe is in place, check for feeling.*)

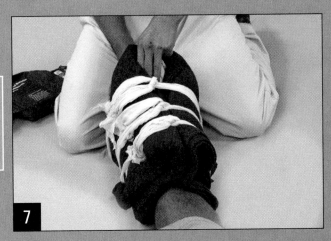

Applying a Rigid Splint

CHECK the scene for safety. **CHECK** the injured person following standard precautions.
CALL 9-1-1 or the local emergency number if necessary. To **CARE** for a person who has an injured limb—

STEP 1
Obtain consent.

STEP 2
Support the injured body part above and below the site of the injury.

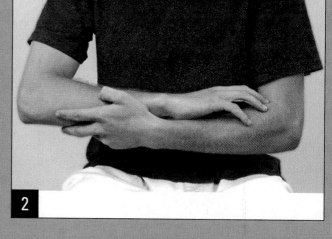

STEP 3
Check for feeling, warmth and color.

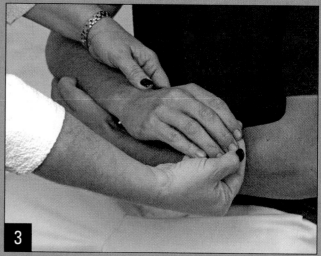

STEP 4

Place the rigid splint (board) under the injured body part and the joints that are above and below the injured body part.

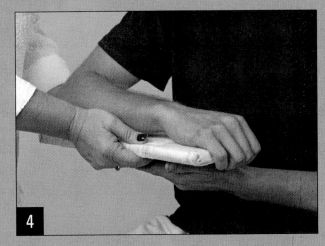

STEP 5

Tie several folded triangular bandages above and below the injured body part.

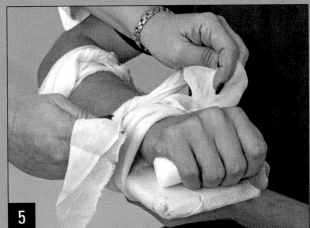

STEP 6

Recheck for feeling, warmth and color.

If a rigid splint is used on an injured forearm, immobilize the wrist and elbow. Bind the arm to the chest using folded triangular bandages or apply a sling.

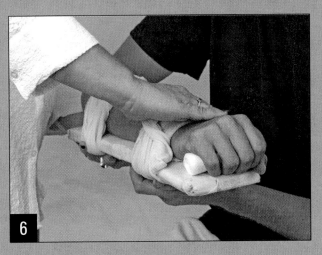

Applying a Sling and Binder

CHECK the scene for safety. **CHECK** the injured person following standard precautions.
CALL 9-1-1 or the local emergency number if necessary. To **CARE** for a person who has an injured limb—

STEP 1
Obtain consent.

STEP 2
Support the injured body part above and below the site of the injury.

STEP 3
Check for feeling, warmth and color.

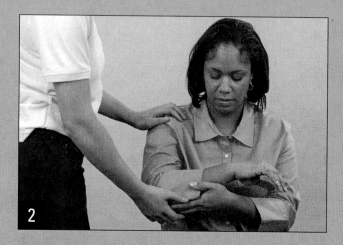

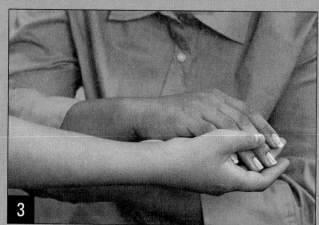

STEP 4

Place a triangular bandage under the injured arm and over the uninjured shoulder to form a sling.

STEP 5

Tie the ends of the sling at the side of the neck.

STEP 6

Bind the injured body part to the chest with a folded triangular bandage.

STEP 7

Recheck for feeling, warmth and color.

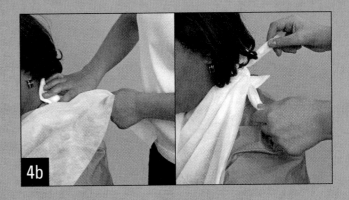

4b

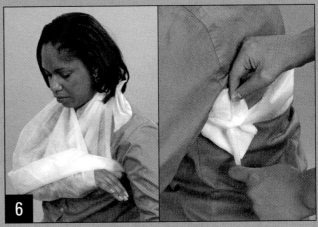

6

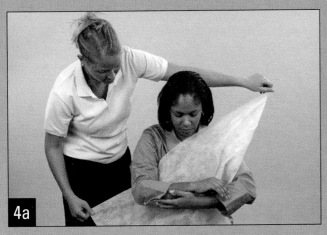

4a

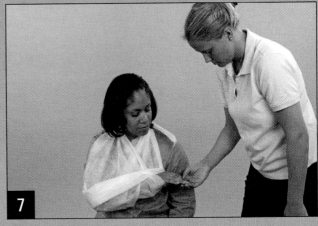

7

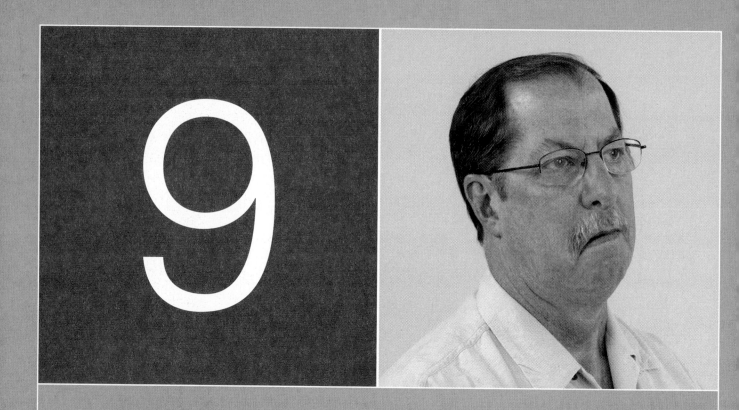

9

If a person becomes suddenly ill, care for any life-threatening conditions first.

Chapter 9

Sudden Illness

It is usually obvious when someone is injured and needs care. The person may be able to tell you what happened and what hurts. Checking the person also gives you clues about what might be wrong. However, when someone becomes suddenly ill, it is not as easy to tell what is wrong. At times there are no signals to give clues about what is happening. At other times, the signals only confirm that something is wrong, without giving additional information. In either case, the signals of a sudden illness often are confusing. You may find it difficult to determine if the person's condition is an emergency and whether to call 9-1-1 or the local emergency number.

RECOGNIZING SUDDEN ILLNESS

When a person becomes suddenly ill, he or she usually looks and feels sick. Common signals include—

- Changes in consciousness, such as feeling lightheaded, dizzy or becoming unconscious.
- Nausea or vomiting.
- Difficulty speaking or slurred speech.
- Numbness or weakness.
- Loss of vision or blurred vision.
- Changes in breathing. The person may have trouble breathing or may not be breathing normally.
- Changes in skin color (pale, ashen or flushed skin).
- Sweating.

- Persistent pressure or pain.
- Diarrhea.
- Seizures.
- Paralysis or inability to move.
- Severe headache.

Besides the physical signals, you may also be able to get clues by looking at the area around the person and finding out what he or she was doing when the illness started. For example, if someone working in a hot environment suddenly becomes ill, it would make sense to suspect the illness is the result of the heat. If someone suddenly feels ill or behaves strangely and is attempting to take medication, the medication may be a clue to what is wrong. For example, the person may take medication for a heart condition, epilepsy or diabetes.

With some sudden illnesses, you might not be sure whether to call 9-1-1 or the local emergency number for help. Sometimes the signals come and go. Remember, if you cannot sort the problem out quickly and easily or if you have any doubts about the severity of the illness, call 9-1-1 or the local emergency number for help.

CARING FOR SUDDEN ILLNESS

Although you probably will not know the exact cause of the sudden illness, you should still give appropriate care.

This is because you will initially care for the signals and not for any specific condition. In the few cases in which you know that the person has a medical condition, such as diabetes, epilepsy or heart disease, the care you give may be slightly different. This care may involve helping the person take medication for his or her specific illness.

Care for sudden illnesses follows the same general guidelines as for any emergency.

- Do no further harm.
- Check the scene for clues about what might be wrong, then check the person.
- Call 9-1-1 or the local emergency number for life-threatening conditions.
- First care for life-threatening conditions such as unconsciousness, trouble breathing, no breathing, no signs of life, severe bleeding, severe chest pain or signals of a stroke, such as weakness, numbness or speech difficulty.
- If the person vomits and is unconscious and lying down, position the person on his or her side.
- Help the person rest comfortably.
- Keep the person from getting chilled or overheated.
- Reassure the person because he or she may be anxious or frightened.
- Watch for changes in consciousness and breathing.
- If the person is conscious, ask if he or she has any medical conditions or is taking any medication.

SPECIFIC SUDDEN ILLNESSES

Fainting

When someone suddenly loses consciousness and then reawakens, he or she may simply have fainted. Fainting is not usually harmful and the person will usually quickly recover. Lower the person to the ground or other flat surface and position him or her on his or her

---

DON'T SECOND GUESS—CALL 9-1-1

Call 9-1-1 or the local emergency number if the person—

- Is unconscious, unusually confused or seems to be losing consciousness.
- Has trouble breathing or is breathing in a strange way.
- Has chest discomfort, pain or pressure that persists for more than 3 to 5 minutes or goes away and comes back.
- Has pressure or discomfort in the abdomen that does not go away.
- Is vomiting blood or passing blood.
- Has a seizure lasting more than 5 minutes or has multiple seizures.
- Has a seizure and is pregnant.
- Has a seizure and is diabetic.
- Has a severe headache or slurred speech or other trouble speaking.
- Has weakness or numbness in his or her body.
- Appears to have been poisoned.
- Has injuries to the head, neck or back.
- Has possible broken bones.

FIGURE 9-1 To care for fainting, place the person on his or her back, elevate the feet and loosen any restrictive clothing, such as a tie or collar.

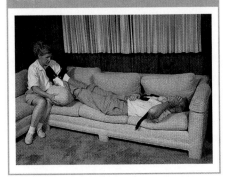

back. If possible, raise the person's legs 8 to 12 inches. Loosen any tight clothing, such as a tie or collar (Fig. 9-1). Check to make sure the person is breathing. Do not give the person anything to eat or drink. If the person vomits, position him or her on one side.

Since you will not be able to tell whether the fainting is a signal of a more serious condition, you should call 9-1-1 or the local emergency number.

Chronic Conditions

Some illnesses that seem to come on suddenly are really caused by chronic conditions. These causes include degenerative diseases, such as heart and lung diseases. There may be a hormone imbalance, such as in diabetes. The person could have epilepsy, a condition that causes seizures. An allergy can cause a sudden and sometimes dangerous reaction to certain substances. When checking a person, look for a medical ID tag, bracelet, necklace or anklet indicating that the person has a chronic condition.

Diabetes

People who are diabetic sometimes become ill because there is too much or too little sugar in their blood. The signals of a diabetic emergency are the same as for any other sudden illness, and they require the same care. You may know the person is a diabetic or the person may tell you he or she is a diabetic. Often diabetics know what is wrong and will ask for something with sugar in it. They may carry some form of sugar with them in case they need it.

If the diabetic person is conscious and can safely swallow food or fluids, give him or her sugar, preferably in liquid form (Fig. 9-2). Most fruit juices and nondiet soft drinks have enough sugar to be effective. You can also give table sugar dissolved in a glass of water. If the person's problem is low blood sugar, sugar will quickly help. If the problem is too much sugar, the sugar will not cause further harm.

Always call 9-1-1 or the local emergency number if—

- The person is unconscious or about to lose consciousness. In this situation, do not give the person anything by mouth. After calling 9-1-1 or the local emergency number, care for the person in the same way as you would care for an unconscious person. This includes making sure the person's airway is clear of vomit and checking breathing and other signs of life until help arrives.

FIGURE 9-2 If the person having a diabetic emergency is conscious and able to swallow, give him or her sugar, preferably in liquid form.

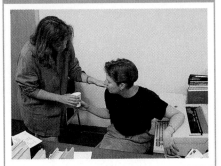

FAINTING

One common signal of sudden illness is a loss of consciousness, such as when a person faints. Fainting is a temporary loss of consciousness. A person who is about to faint often becomes pale, begins to sweat and then loses consciousness and collapses.

Fainting occurs when there is an insufficient supply of blood to the brain for a short period of time. This condition results from a widening of the blood vessels in the body, which causes blood to drain away from the brain. A person who feels weak or dizzy may prevent a fainting spell by lying down or sitting with the head level with the knees.

A person who has fainted usually will recover quickly with no lasting effects. But what appears to be a simple case of fainting may actually be a signal of a more serious condition. If a serious condition is suspected or an injury occurs, call 9-1-1 or the local emergency number. However, it may be appropriate to take the person to a physician or emergency department to determine if the fainting episode is linked to a more serious condition.

DIABETES: A SILENT KILLER

More than 18 million people in the United States have diabetes. Among this group, more than 5 million people are unaware that they have the disease. Diabetes was the sixth-leading cause of death listed on U.S. death certificates in 2000. Altogether, diabetes contributed to 213,062 deaths. Diabetes is likely to be underreported as a cause of death. Overall, the risk for death among people with diabetes is about twice that of people without diabetes.

Diabetes can lead to other medical conditions such as blindness, nerve disease, kidney disease, heart disease and stroke. The American Diabetes Association defines diabetes as the inability of the body to convert sugar from food into energy.

The cells in your body need sugar as a source of energy. The cells receive this energy during digestion, when the body breaks food into sugars. The sugar then becomes absorbed into the blood with the help of a hormone called *insulin*. Insulin is produced in the body and takes sugar into the cells. For the body to function properly, there has to be a balance of insulin and sugar in the body or the cells will starve.

When insulin is not produced or used in the proper amount, diabetes occurs. There are two major types of diabetes: Type I, insulin-dependent diabetes, and Type II, non-insulin-dependent diabetes. Diabetes is a chronic disease that currently has no cure.

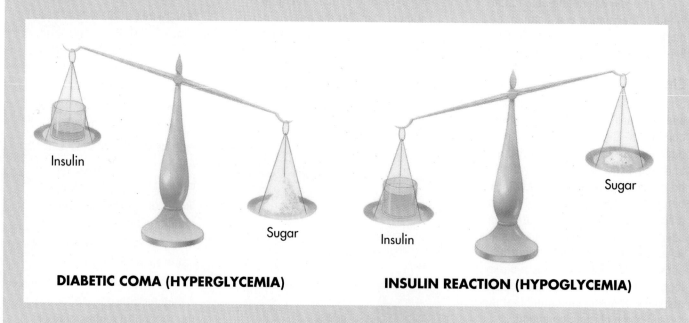

Insulin   Sugar

DIABETIC COMA (HYPERGLYCEMIA)

Insulin   Sugar

INSULIN REACTION (HYPOGLYCEMIA)

Type I diabetes, also called juvenile diabetes, affects about 1 million Americans. This type of diabetes, which usually begins in childhood, occurs when the body produces little or no insulin. People with Type I diabetes must inject insulin into their bodies daily, and are therefore considered to be insulin-dependent.

The exact cause of Type I diabetes is not known. Warning signals include—
• Frequent urination.
• Increased hunger and thirst.
• Unexpected weight loss.
• Irritability.
• Weakness and fatigue.

Type II diabetes, also called adult-onset diabetes, is the most common type. It affects about 90 to 95 percent of people with diabetes. This condition usually occurs in adults, but also can occur in children—mostly those who are overweight. With Type II diabetes, the body makes insulin but not enough for what the body needs. In some cases of Type II diabetes, the body becomes resistant to the insulin produced. People with this type of diabetes are considered non-insulin-dependent.

According to the American Diabetes Association, "Medical experts do not know the exact cause of Type II diabetes. They do know Type II diabetes runs in families. A person can inherit a tendency to get Type II diabetes, but it usually takes another factor, such as obesity, to bring on the disease."

Individuals from certain racial and ethnic backgrounds are known to be at greater risk for diabetes. Type II diabetes is more common among African-Americans, Latinos, Asians, certain Native Americans and Pacific Islanders.

Warning signals of Type II diabetes include—
• Any signals of Type I diabetes.
• Frequent infections, especially involving the skin, gums and bladder.
• Blurred vision.
• Numbness in legs, feet and fingers.
• Cuts/bruises that are slow to heal.
• Itching.

People with Type II diabetes often have no signals.

It is important for anyone with diabetes to monitor his or her exercise and diet. Self-monitoring for blood sugar levels is a valuable tool. Insulin-dependent diabetics must also monitor their use of insulin. If a diabetic does not control these factors, an imbalance between insulin and sugar in the body can create a diabetic emergency. Signals of a diabetic emergency include—
• Changes in the level of consciousness.
• Rapid breathing and pulse.
• Feeling and looking ill.

For more information about diabetes, contact the American Diabetes Association at 1-800-DIABETES or *www.diabetes.org*

For specific information about Type I diabetes, contact the Juvenile Diabetes Foundation at 1-800-JDF-CURE or at *info@jdf.org*

- The person is conscious and unable to swallow. (In this case, do not put anything, liquid or solid, into the person's mouth.)
- The person does not feel better within about 5 minutes after taking sugar.
- You cannot find sugar immediately. Do not spend time looking for it.

Seizures

Sometimes a person who becomes suddenly ill may have a seizure. Although it may be frightening to watch, you can easily help care for the person. Remember that he or she cannot control the seizure. Do not try to stop the seizure. Do not hold or restrain the person, nor put anything in the person's mouth.

Care for a person who has had a seizure the same way you would for an unconscious person. To protect the person from being injured, remove nearby objects that might cause injury. Protect the person's head by placing a thin cushion under it. Folded clothing makes an adequate cushion. If there is fluid in the person's mouth, such as saliva, blood or vomit, roll him or her on one side so that the fluid drains from the mouth.

Do not try to place anything between the person's teeth. People having seizures rarely bite their tongues or cheeks with enough force to cause significant bleeding. However, some blood may be present.

When the seizure is over, the person will usually begin to breathe normally. He or she may be drowsy and disoriented or unresponsive for a period of time. Check to see if the person was injured during the seizure. Be reassuring and comforting. If the seizure occurred in public, the person may be embarrassed and self-conscious. Ask bystanders not to crowd around the person. He or she will be tired and want to rest. Stay with the person until he or she

---

DID YOU KNOW?

SEIZURES

When the normal workings of the brain are disrupted by injury, disease, fever or infection, the electrical activity of the brain becomes irregular. This can cause a loss of body control known as a *seizure.* Seizures may be caused by extreme heat, a diabetic condition or an injury to the brain.

Seizures may be caused by an acute or chronic condition. The chronic condition is known as *epilepsy.* Over 2 million Americans have epilepsy. Epilepsy is usually controlled with medication. Still, some people with epilepsy have seizures from time to time. Others who go a long time without a seizure may think the condition has gone away and stop taking their medication. These people may then have a seizure again.

A person with epilepsy may experience something called an *aura* before the seizure occurs. An aura is an unusual sensation or feeling such as a visual hallucination; strange sound, taste or smell; or an urgent need to get to safety. If the person recognizes the aura, he or she may have time to tell bystanders and sit down before the seizure occurs.

Seizures range from a blank stare or period of distorted sensation during which the person is unable to respond to sudden, uncontrolled muscular contractions called *convulsions,* which last several minutes. Infants and young children are at risk for seizures brought on by high fever. These are called *febrile* (heat-induced) *seizures.*

Although it may be frightening to see someone unexpectedly having a seizure, you should remember that most seizures last only for a few minutes and the person usually recovers without problems.

is fully conscious and aware of the surroundings.

If the person is known to have occasional seizures, you do not have to call 9-1-1 or the local emergency number. He or she will usually recover from a seizure in a few minutes. However, call 9-1-1 or the local emergency number if—

- The seizure lasts more than 5 minutes.
- The person has multiple seizures.
- The person appears to be injured.
- The person is pregnant.
- The person is a diabetic.
- The seizure follows a quick rise in the person's temperature.
- The person fails to regain consciousness.

Having to deal with a sudden illness can be scary, especially when you do not know what is wrong. Do not hesitate to give care. Remember, you do not have to know the cause to help. As you can see, the signals for sudden illnesses are very similar to other conditions and the care involves skills that you already know.

STROKE

Stroke is the third-leading killer in the United States, and is the number one reason why people are admitted to nursing homes. About 700,000 Americans will have a stroke this year.

A *stroke,* also called a "brain attack," is caused when blood flow to a part of the brain is cut off, or when there is bleeding into the brain. Strokes can cause permanent brain damage, but sometimes the damage can be stopped or reversed.

A stroke usually is caused by a blockage in the arteries that supply blood to the brain. Once the blood flow is cut off, that part of the brain starts to "suffocate" and die, unless the blood flow can be restored. Blockages can be caused by blood clots, which

travel from other parts of the body, like the heart, or they can be caused by slow damage to the arteries over time from high blood pressure and diabetes, for example.

In about 20 percent of strokes there is bleeding into the brain. This bleeding can be from a broken blood vessel or from a bulging aneurysm that breaks open. There is no way to tell if someone is having a bleeding type stroke from a blocked artery type of stroke until they get to the emergency room and get X-rays of their head.

A "mini-stroke" is when a person has the signals of a stroke, which then completely go away. Most mini-strokes, or transient ischemic attacks (TIAs) get better within a few minutes, although they can last several hours. Although the signals of a mini-stroke disappear quickly, the person is not out of danger at that point. In fact, someone who has a mini-stroke is at very high risk of having a full-blown stroke in the next 2 days. Mini-strokes should be considered an emergency, too, even if the signals have gone away, and you should call 9-1-1 or the local emergency number.

Risk Factors

A stroke can be caused by a blood clot or bleeding from a ruptured artery in the brain.

The risk factors for stroke, meaning things that make a stroke more likely, are similar to those for heart disease. Some risk factors are beyond your control, such as older age, male gender, family history of stroke, previous mini-stroke, diabetes or heart disease. However, even if you do not have these risk factors, it is still possible that you can have a stroke. Some risk factors are within your ability to control, including high blood pressure, cigarette smoking and diet.

High Blood Pressure. If you have high blood pressure, you are approximately seven times more likely to have a stroke than is someone who does not have high blood pressure.

High blood pressure puts pressure on arteries and makes them stiffer. The pressure then goes downstream and damages your organs, including your brain, heart, kidneys, etc. Even mildly high blood pressure can increase your risk of stroke. Have your blood pressure checked regularly and, if it is high, follow your physician's advice on how to lower it. You can often control high blood pressure by losing weight, changing your diet, exercising routinely and managing stress. If those measures are not sufficient, your physician may prescribe medication.

Cigarette Smoking. Cigarette smoking is another major risk factor of stroke. Smoking is linked to heart disease and cancer, as well as to stroke. Smoking increases blood pressure, damages blood vessels and makes blood more likely to clot. If you smoke and would like to quit, many techniques and support systems are available to help, including your physician and local health department.

The benefits of not smoking begin as soon as you stop, and some of smoking's damage may actually be reversible. Approximately 10 years after a person has stopped smoking, his or her risk of stroke is the same as the risk for a person who has never smoked. Even if you do not smoke, be aware that inhaling smoke from smokers can harm your health. Avoid long-term exposure to cigarette smoke and protect children from this danger as well.

Diet. Diets that are high in saturated fats and cholesterol can increase your risk of stroke by causing fatty materials to build up on the walls of your blood vessels. Foods high in choles-

FAST RECOGNITION OF STROKE

For a stroke, think **FAST!**

- **F**ace—Weakness on one side of the face (Fig. 9-3, A).
  - ○ Ask the person to smile. This will show if there is drooping or weakness in the muscles on one side of the face.

- **A**rm—Weakness or numbness in one arm (Fig. 9-3, B).
  - ○ Ask the person to raise both arms to find out if there is weakness in the limbs.

- **S**peech—Slurred speech or trouble speaking.
  - ○ Ask the person to speak a simple sentence to listen for slurred or distorted speech. Example: "I have the lunch orders ready."

- **T**ime—Time to **CALL 9-1-1** or the local emergency number if you see any of these signals.
  - ○ Note the time that the signals began and call 9-1-1 or the local emergency number right away.

FIGURE 9-3, A-B

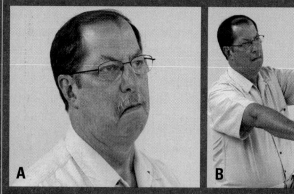
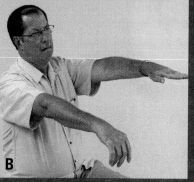

A   B

The FAST mnemonic is based on the Cincinnati Pre-Hospital Stroke Scale, which was originally developed for emergency medical services (EMS) workers in 1997. The scale was designed to help paramedics identify strokes in the field, so that they can prepare the emergency room before they arrive. The FAST method for public awareness has been in use in the community in Cincinnati, Ohio since 1999, and has since been used in several other variations of the message. It was validated by researchers at the University of North Carolina in 2003.

terol include egg yolks and organ meats, such as liver and kidneys. Saturated fats are found in beef, lamb, veal, pork, ham, whole milk and whole-milk products. Limiting your intake of these foods can help prevent stroke.

Diabetes. Diabetes is another major risk factor for stroke. If you have been diagnosed with diabetes, follow your physician's advice about how to control it. If uncontrolled, the high blood sugar of diabetes can cause damage to blood vessels throughout the body.

By paying attention to the signals of stroke and reporting them to your physician, you can prevent damage before it occurs. Experiencing a mini-stroke is the clearest warning that a stroke may occur. Do not ignore its stroke-like signals, even if they disappear completely within minutes or hours.

Stroke Prevention

You can help prevent stroke if you—
- Control your blood pressure.
- Do not smoke.
- Eat a healthy diet.
- Exercise regularly.
- Control diabetes.

Regular exercise reduces your chances of stroke by strengthening the heart and improving blood circulation. Exercise also helps in weight control. Being overweight increases the chance of developing high blood pressure, heart disease and fat deposits lining the arteries.

Sudden Signals of a Stroke

As with other sudden illnesses, the primary signals of a stroke or mini-stroke are a sudden change in how the body is working or feeling. This usually includes sudden weakness or numbness of the face, arm or leg. Usually, weakness or numbness occurs only on one side of the body. In addition, the person may—
- Have difficulty talking or being understood when speaking.
- Have blurred or dimmed vision.

- Experience a sudden, severe headache; dizziness; or confusion.

Care for a Stroke

If you encounter someone who is having or has had a stroke, call 9-1-1 or the local emergency number immediately. Look at your watch and note the time the signals started. If the person is unconscious, make sure that he or she has an open airway and care for life-threatening conditions. If fluid or vomit is in the person's mouth, position him or her on one side to allow fluids to drain out of the mouth.

Stay with the person and monitor his or her breathing and other signs of life. If the person is conscious, check for nonlife-threatening conditions. If you see signals of a stroke, call 9-1-1 or the local emergency number immediately. A stroke can make the person fearful and anxious. Often, he or she does not understand what has happened. Offer comfort and reassurance. Have the person rest in a comfortable position. Do not give him or her anything to eat or drink.

In the past, a stroke almost always caused irreversible brain damage. Today, new medications and medical procedures can limit or reduce the damage caused by stroke. Many of these new treatments must be given quickly to be effective. Therefore, you should immediately call 9-1-1 or the local emergency number to get the best care.

[handwritten notes:]
F ACE — SMILE
A RM — EXTEND + RAISE
S AY — SLURRED SPEECH
T — TIME (NOTE + DESCRIBE TO 911)

THROMBOLYTIC DRUGS, OR "CLOT-BUSTERS"

Used to treat an ongoing stroke with a blocked artery (ischemic), these drugs halt the stroke by dissolving the blood clot that is blocking blood flow to the brain. *Recombinant tissue plasminogen activator (rt-PA),* for example, is approved by the Food and Drug Administration (FDA) to treat strokes, but only those that come to a hospital extremely quickly. If given quickly and correctly, people who receive this medicine are 55 percent more likely to go home than to a nursing home. Unfortunately, these medicines only work if given within a few hours after signals begin, which is why knowing when the signals began and calling 9-1-1 are so important in stroke patients.

Much research is being conducted to find different drugs or devices to treat ischemic stroke, and also to try and lengthen the time window so more people may receive treatment. While many trials are underway, none of these other drugs has been approved by the FDA. One other device has been approved by the FDA in patients who do not qualify for the clot-buster drug. It is called the Merci device. This tiny device is threaded through an artery in the groin and up into the brain. Once the blood clot is found, the device, which looks like a corkscrew, is put into the catheter and the blood clot is pulled back out of the brain. This is still being studied. Other trials are underway studying different ways of giving the clot-buster drugs. For instance, one trial gives some medicine through the vein, and some through the catheter threaded up into the brain.

CARE FOR SUDDEN ILLNESS

Care for life-threatening conditions first. Then—
- Help the person rest comfortably.
- Keep the person from getting chilled or overheated.
- Reassure the person.
- Watch for changes in consciousness and breathing.
- Do not give anything to eat or drink unless the person is fully conscious and does not have a droopy face on one side or slurred speech.

If the person—
- Vomits—Place him or her on one side so that you can clear the mouth.
- Faints—Position him or her on the back and elevate the legs 8 to 12 inches if you do not suspect a head, neck or back injury.
- Has a diabetic emergency—Give the conscious person who is able to swallow some type of sugar, preferably in liquid form, such as orange or apple juice, nondiet soda or 2 to 3 teaspoons of sugar dissolved in a glass of water.
- Has a seizure—Do not hold or restrain the person or place anything between the person's teeth. Remove any nearby objects that might cause injury. Cushion the person's head using folded clothing or a small pillow.
- Has a severe allergic reaction—Assist the person with his or her medication, which may be available as a single-dose epinephrine auto-injector.

10

About 92 percent of all poisonings take place in the home.

Chapter 10

Poisoning

A poison is any substance that causes injury, illness or death if it enters the body. A person can be poisoned by swallowing poison, breathing it, absorbing it through the skin and by having it injected into the body.

In 2002, Poison Control Centers received more than 2.3 million calls having to do with people who had come into contact with a poison. In 2003, about 92 percent of all poisonings took place in the home and 52 percent involved children under the age of 6 years. Poisoning deaths in children under age 6 represented about 3 percent of the total deaths from poisoning, while the 20- to 49-year-old age group represented 58 percent of all deaths from poisoning.

In recent years there has been a decrease in child poisonings, due in part to childproof packaging for medications, which makes it harder for children to get into these substances. The decrease is also a result of preventive actions by parents and others who care for children. At the same time, there has been an increase in adult poisoning deaths, which is linked to an increase in both suicides and drug-related poisonings.

SWALLOWED, INHALED, ABSORBED AND INJECTED POISONS

Swallowed Poisons

Poisons that can be swallowed include foods, such as certain mushrooms and shellfish; drugs, such as sleeping pills, tranquilizers and alcohol; medications, such as aspirin; household items, such as cleaning products and pesticides; and certain plants (Fig. 10-1, A). Many substances not poisonous in small amounts are poisonous in larger amounts. Combinations of certain substances can be poisonous if taken together, although if taken by themselves they might not cause harm.

Inhaled Poisons

A person can be poisoned by breathing in (inhaling) toxic fumes (Fig. 10-1, B). Examples of poisons that can be inhaled include—

- Gases, such as—
  - Carbon monoxide from an engine or car exhaust.
  - Carbon dioxide from wells and sewers.
  - Chlorine, found in many swimming pools.
- Fumes from—
  - Household products, such as glues and paints.
  - Drugs, such as crack cocaine.

DID YOU KNOW?

SUBSTANCE ABUSE

Numerous drugs and other substances are abused in our society, with a wide range of psychological and physical effects. Signals of possible substance abuse include—

- Behavioral changes not otherwise explained.
- Sudden mood changes.
- Restlessness, talkativeness, irritability.
- Altered consciousness.
- Slurred speech, poor coordination.
- Moist or flushed skin.
- Chills, nausea, vomiting.
- Dizziness, confusion.
- Irregular pulse.
- Irregular breathing.
- Loss of consciousness.

What to Do

If you think the person took an overdose or has another substance abuse problem requiring medical attention or other professional help, you should check the scene for safety and check the person. If you have good reason to suspect a substance was taken, call the National Poison Control Center (800-222-1222) and follow the call taker's directions.

Call 9-1-1 or the local emergency number if the person—

- Is unconscious, confused or seems to be losing consciousness.
- Has trouble breathing or is breathing irregularly.
- Has persistent chest pain or pressure.
- Has pressure or pain in the abdomen that does not go away.
- Is vomiting blood or passing blood.
- Has a seizure, severe headache or slurred speech.
- Acts violently.

Also call 9-1-1 or the local emergency number if you are unsure what to do or you are unsure about the severity of the problem.

Care for Substance Abuse

To care for the person, you should—

- Try to learn from others what substances may have been taken.
- Calm and reassure the person.
- Keep the person from getting chilled or overheated to minimize shock.

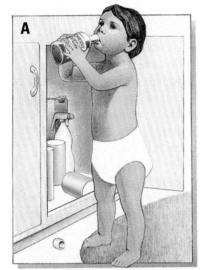

Ingestion

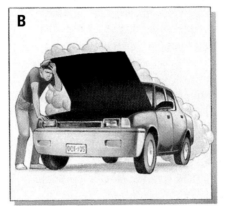

Inhalation

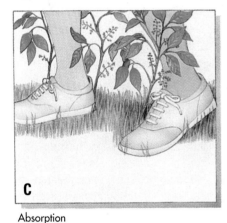

C

Absorption

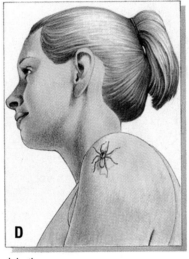

D

Injection

PREVENTING POISONING WITH COMMON SENSE

Use common sense when handling substances that could be harmful, such as chemicals and cleaners. Use them in a well-ventilated area. Wear protective clothing, such as gloves and a face mask.

Use common sense with your own medications. Read the product information and use only as directed. Ask your health-care provider or pharmacist about the intended effects, side effects and possible interactions with other medications you are taking. Never use another person's prescribed medications. What is right for one person is seldom right for another.

Always keep medications in the containers they came in and make sure the container is well marked. Destroy all out-of-date medications by disposing of the contents in the toilet. Over time they can become less effective and even toxic.

Absorbed Poisons

Poisons that can be absorbed through the skin come from many sources including plants, such as poison ivy, poison oak and poison sumac, and fertilizers and pesticides (Fig. 10-1, C).

Injected Poisons

Injected poisons enter the body through the bites or stings of insects, spiders, ticks, some marine life, snakes and other animals or through drugs or medications injected with a hypodermic needle (Fig. 10-1, D).

CHECKING THE SCENE FOR POISONING

How will you know if someone who is ill has been poisoned? Look for clues about what has happened. Try to get information from the person or from bystanders. As you check the scene, be aware of unusual odors, flames, smoke, open or spilled containers, an open medicine cabinet, an overturned or a damaged plant. Also notice if the person is showing any of the following signals of poisoning:

- Nausea and vomiting
- Diarrhea
- Chest or abdominal pain
- Trouble breathing
- Sweating
- Changes in consciousness
- Seizures
- Headache
- Dizziness
- Weakness
- Irregular pupil size

- Burning or tearing eyes
- Abnormal skin color
- Burns around the lips, tongue or on the skin

You may also suspect a poisoning based on information you have from or about the person. If you suspect someone has swallowed a poison, try to find out—

- The type of poison.
- The quantity taken.
- When it was taken.
- How much the person weighs.

This information can help you and others give the most appropriate care.

GENERAL CARE FOR POISONING

After you have checked the scene and determined that there has been a poisoning, follow these general care guidelines:

- Remove the person from the source of poison if the scene is dangerous.
- Check the person's level of consciousness, breathing and other signs of life.
- Care for any life-threatening conditions.
- If the person is conscious, ask questions to get more information.
- Look for any containers and take them with you to the telephone.
- Call the National Poison Control Center (800-222-1222), 9-1-1 or the local emergency number.
- Follow the directions of the Poison Control Center or the emergency medical services (EMS) call taker.

If the person becomes violent or threatening, retreat to safety and wait for help to arrive. Do not give the person anything to eat or drink unless medical professionals tell you to do so. If you do not know what the poison was and the person vomits, save some of the vomit. The hospital may analyze it to identify the poison.

SPECIAL CARE CONSIDERATIONS

Toxic Fumes

It is often difficult to tell if a poisoning victim has inhaled toxic fumes. Toxic fumes come from a variety of sources. They may have an odor or be odor-free. When someone breathes in toxic fumes, the person's skin may turn pale or ashen. This may indicate a lack of oxygen. If it is safe for you to do so, get the person to fresh air. Anyone who has inhaled toxic fumes needs fresh air as soon as possible.

Wet and Dry Chemicals

If poisons such as wet chemicals get on the skin, flush the affected area with large amounts of cool water (Fig. 10-2). Have someone else call 9-1-1 or the local emergency number. Keep flushing the area until EMS personnel arrive.

Brush off dry chemicals, such as lime, with gloved hands and then flush the area thoroughly with large amounts of cool water. Take care not to get any in your eyes or the eyes of the person or of bystanders.

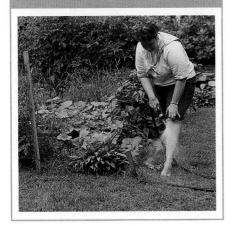

FIGURE 10-2 If poisons such as wet chemicals get on the skin, flush the affected area with large amounts of cool water.

Insects

Insect stings are painful, but they are rarely fatal. Some people, however, have a severe allergic reaction to an insect sting. This allergic reaction may result in a breathing emergency.

If someone is stung by an insect—
- Remove the stinger. Scrape it away from the skin with your fingernail or a plastic card, such as a credit card, or use tweezers (Fig. 10-3). If you use tweezers, grasp the stinger, not the venom sac.
- Wash the site with soap and water.

- Cover the site and keep it clean.
- Apply a cold pack to the area to reduce pain and swelling.
- Watch the person for signals of an allergic reaction.

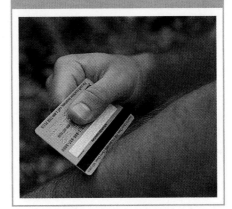

FIGURE 10-3 If someone is stung by an insect, remove the stinger. Scrape it away from the skin with your fingernail or a plastic card, such as a credit card.

Scorpions and Spiders

Scorpions live in dry regions of the southwestern United States under rocks, logs and the bark of certain trees (Fig. 10-4). They are most active at night. Only a few species of scorpions have a sting that can cause death.

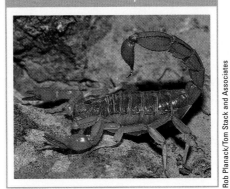

FIGURE 10-4 Scorpion.

Rob Planack/Tom Stack and Associates

Only two spiders in the United States—the black widow and the brown recluse—have a bite that can kill or seriously injure (Fig. 10-5, A-B). The black widow spider is black with a reddish hourglass shape on the underside of its body. Both spiders prefer dark, out-of-the-way places. They usually bite the hands and arms of people who are reaching into places such as wood, rock and brush piles or rummaging in dark garages and attics. Often, the person will not know that he or she has been bitten until he or

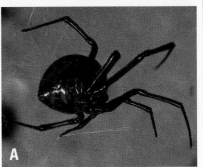

FIGURE 10-5, A-B Bites from the A, black widow spider and the B, brown recluse spider can make you sick or be fatal.

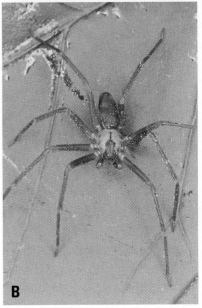

Rob Planack/Tom Stack and Associates

Ann Moreton/Tom Stack and Associates

LYME DISEASE

Lyme disease, an illness that people get from the bite of an infected tick, is affecting a growing number of people in the United States. Although Lyme disease has been reported in almost every state, 90 percent of the cases reported in the past decade have been in 10 states: New York, Connecticut, Pennsylvania, New Jersey, Wisconsin, Rhode Island, Maryland, Massachusetts, Minnesota and Delaware. Because Lyme disease appears to be spreading, everyone should take precautions to protect against it.

Not all ticks carry Lyme disease. Lyme disease is spread mainly by a type of tick sometimes called the *deer tick*, which often attaches itself to field mice and deer. The tick is found around branches and in wooded and grassy areas. Like all ticks, it attaches itself to any warm-blooded animal that brushes by it, including humans. A deer tick can attach to you without your knowledge. Many people who develop Lyme disease cannot recall having been bitten.

The Tiniest of Ticks

Deer ticks are tiny and difficult to see. They are much smaller than the common dog tick or wood tick. They can be as small as a poppy seed or the head of a pin. Adult deer ticks are only as large as a grape seed. Because of the tick's tiny size, its bite is usually painless.

You can get Lyme disease from the bite of an infected tick at any time of the year. In northern states, however, the risk is greatest between May and late August, when ticks are most active and people spend more time outdoors. Recent studies indicate that the tick must remain embedded in human skin for about 48 hours to transmit Lyme disease.

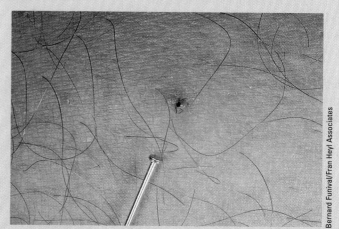

A deer tick can be as small as the head of a pin.

Signals of Lyme Disease

The first signal of infection may appear a few days or a few weeks after a tick bite. Typically, a rash starts as a small red area at the site of the bite. It may spread up to 7 inches across. In fair-skinned people, the center is lighter in color and the outer edges are red and raised. This sometimes gives the rash a bull's-eye appearance. In dark-skinned people, the area may look black and blue, like a bruise.

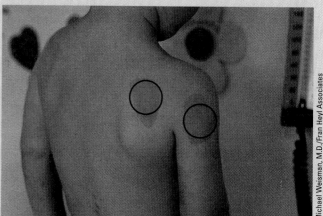

A person with Lyme disease may develop a rash.

Other signals of Lyme disease include fever, headache, weakness and joint and muscle pain similar to the signals of flu. These signals can develop slowly and might not occur at the same time as the rash. Some people with Lyme disease never develop a rash.

Lyme disease can get worse if not treated. In its advanced stages it may cause arthritis, numbness, memory loss, problems in seeing or hearing, high fever and stiff neck. Some of these signals could indicate problems with the brain or nervous system. An irregular or rapid heartbeat could indicate heart problems.

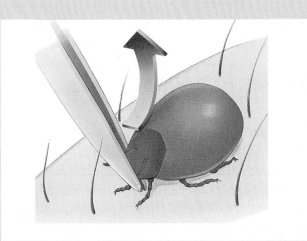

Remove a tick by pulling slowly, steadily and firmly with a pair of fine-tipped tweezers.

Preventing Lyme Disease

To prevent Lyme disease, always check for ticks immediately after outdoor activities. Wash all clothing. Be sure to check pets because they can develop signals of Lyme disease as well as carry ticks into the house, where they can then attach themselves to unsuspecting people or other pets.

If you find a tick, remove it by pulling steadily and firmly. Grasp the tick with fine-tipped tweezers, as close to the skin as possible, and pull slowly. If you do not have tweezers, use a glove, plastic wrap or a piece of paper to protect your fingers. If you use your bare fingers, wash your hands immediately. Do not try to burn a tick off with a hot match or burning cigarette. Do not use other home remedies, such as coating the tick with petroleum jelly or nail polish or pricking it with a pin.

Once the tick is removed, wash the area immediately with soap and water. If an antiseptic or triple antibiotic ointment is available, apply it to prevent infection. Check the site from time to time to see if it has become infected.

If you cannot remove the tick or if parts of the tick stay in your skin, seek medical care. Also seek medical care if a rash or flu-like signals develop. A physician will usually prescribe antibiotics to treat Lyme disease. Antibiotics work best and most quickly when taken early. If you suspect Lyme disease, do not delay seeking treatment. Treatment is slower and less effective in advanced stages.

More information on Lyme disease may be available from your local or state health department. Be sure to ask about current recommendations for the Lyme disease vaccine.

For information about other tick-borne diseases, visit the Centers for Disease Control and Prevention (CDC) Web site at *www.cdc.gov/ncidod/ diseases/insects/diseases.htm*

WEST NILE VIRUS: WHAT YOU NEED TO KNOW

In recent years, West Nile Virus (WNV) has been reported in some mild areas of North America and Europe. WNV is passed on to humans and other animals by mosquitoes that bite them after feeding on infected birds.

About one in every 150 people who are infected with WNV will become seriously ill. Signals can include high fever, headache, neck stiffness, confusion, coma, tremors, convulsions, muscle weakness, vision loss, numbness and paralysis. These signals may last several weeks. In some cases, WNV can cause fatal encephalitis, which is a swelling of the brain that leads to death.

Most people infected with WNV have no signals. Approximately 20 percent develop mild signals, such as fever and aches, which pass on their own. The risk of severe disease is higher for people 50 years of age and older. People typically develop signals between 3 and 14 days after they are bitten by an infected mosquito.

WNV cannot be passed from one person to another, and there is no evidence that a person can become infected by handling live or dead infected birds. However, it is still a good idea to use a protective barrier, such as plastic gloves, if you are going to handle an infected bird. Contact your local health department for instructions on reporting and disposing of the bird's body.

There is no specific treatment for WNV infection or vaccine to prevent it. In more severe cases, people usually need to go to the hospital where they can receive treatment, including intravenous fluids, help with breathing and nursing care.

If you develop signals of severe WNV illness, such as unusually severe headaches or confusion, seek medical attention immediately. Pregnant women and nursing mothers are encouraged to talk to their doctor if they develop signals that could be WNV.

Risks of Catching WNV

For most people, the risk of catching WNV is very low. Less than 1 percent of people who are bitten by mosquitoes develop any signals of the disease and relatively few mosquitoes actually carry WNV. Pregnancy and nursing do not increase the risk of becoming infected. The risk of getting WNV through blood transfusions, and organ transplants is very small. The one group with a somewhat higher risk for catching the disease is people who spend a lot of time outdoors.

Preventing WNV

The easiest and best way to avoid WNV is to prevent mosquito bites. Specifically, you can—

- Use insect repellents containing DEET (N, N-diethyl-meta-toluamide) when you are outdoors. Follow the directions on the package.
- Consider staying indoors at dusk and dawn when mosquitoes are most active. If you have to be outdoors during these times, use insect repellent and wear long sleeves and pants. Light-colored clothing can help you see mosquitoes that land on you.
- Make sure you have good screens on your windows and doors to keep mosquitoes out.
- Get rid of mosquito breeding sites by emptying standing water from flower pots, buckets and barrels. For example, change the water in pet dishes and replace the water in bird baths weekly, drill drainage holes in tire swings so water drains out and keep children's wading pools empty and on their sides when they aren't being used.

For more information, visit *www.cdc.gov/westnile*, or call the CDC public response hotline at (888) 246-2675 (English), (888) 246-2857 (Español), or (866) 874-2646 (TTY).

Source: *CDC.gov* and *redcross.org*

she starts to feel ill or notices a bite mark or swelling.

Signals of spider bites and scorpion stings also are similar to those of other sudden illnesses. In addition, the person might salivate more than normal, experience severe pain and swelling around the sting or bite, and have a mark indicating where the sting or bite occurred.

If you encounter someone who might have been bitten by a scorpion, a black widow or brown recluse—

- Wash the wound.
- Apply a cold pack to the site.
- Call 9-1-1 or the local emergency number.
- If it is available, give the person antivenin—a medication that blocks the effects of the spider's poisonous venom.

Snakes

Snakebites kill very few people in the United States. Of the estimated 7000 people bitten annually, fewer than five die (Fig. 10-6, A-D). Most snakebites occur near the home, not in the wild. Rattlesnakes account for most snakebites and nearly all of the deaths from snakebites in the United States. Most deaths occur because the bitten person has an allergic reaction, is in poor health or because too much time passes before he or she receives medical care.

Care for Snakebites. To care for a bite from a pit viper, such as a rattlesnake, copperhead or cottonmouth, follow these steps:

- Call 9-1-1 or the local emergency number.
- Wash the wound.
- Keep the injured area still and lower than the heart. If possible, carry a person who must be taken to a medical facility or have him or her walk slowly.
- **DO NOT** Apply ice.
- **DO NOT** Cut the wound.
- **DO NOT** Apply suction.

FIGURE 10-6, A-D There are four kinds of poisonous snakes found in the United States: A, Rattlesnake B, Copperhead C, Cottonmouth D, Coral snake.

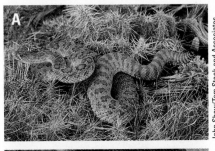
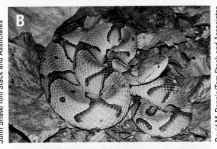
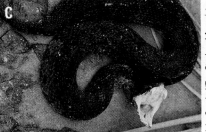
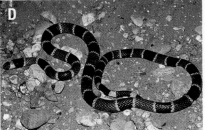

- **DO NOT** Apply a tourniquet.
- **DO NOT** Use electric shock, such as from a car battery.

Care for a bite from an elapid snake, such as a coral snake, is the same as for a pit viper, except that after washing the wound you should apply an elastic roller bandage by fol-lowing these steps (see Chapter 7 for more information):

- Check the circulation (feeling, warmth and color) of the limb beyond where you will be placing the bandage by noting changes in skin color and temperature.
- Place the end of the bandage against the skin and use over-lapping turns.

- Gently stretch the bandage as you continue wrapping. The wrap should cover a long body section, such as an arm or a calf, begin-ning at the point farthest from the heart. For a joint like a knee or ankle, use figure-eight turns to support the joint.
- Always check the area above and below the injury site for feeling, warmth and color, especially fin-gers and toes, after you have applied an elastic roller bandage. By checking before and after bandaging, you will be able to tell if any tingling or numbness is from the bandaging or the injury.
- Check the snugness of the band-aging—a finger should easily, but not loosely, pass under the bandage.
- Keep the injured area still and lower than the heart. If possible, carry a person who must be taken to a medical facility or have him or her walk slowly.
- **DO NOT** Apply ice.
- **DO NOT** Cut the wound.
- **DO NOT** Apply suction.
- **DO NOT** Apply a tourniquet.
- **DO NOT** Use electric shock, such as from a car battery.

Animals

The bite of a domestic or wild animal can cause infection and soft tissue injury. The most serious possible result is rabies. Rabies is transmitted through the saliva of diseased animals such as skunks, bats, raccoons, cats, dogs, cattle and foxes.

Animals with rabies may act strangely. For example, those that are usually active at night may be active in the daytime. A wild animal that usually tries to avoid people might not run from you. Rabid animals may drool, appear partially paralyzed or act irrita-ble, mean or strangely quiet.

If not treated, rabies is fatal. Any-one bitten by an animal that might

HOW TO BEAT THOSE LITTLE CRITTERS

You can prevent bites and stings from insects, spiders, ticks or snakes by following these guidelines when you are in wooded or grassy areas:

- Wear long-sleeved shirts and long pants.
- Tuck your pant legs into your socks or boots.
- Use a rubber band or tape to hold pants against socks so that nothing can get under clothing.
- Tuck your shirt into your pants.
- Wear light-colored clothing to make it easier to see tiny insects or ticks.
- When hiking in woods and fields, stay in the middle of trails. Avoid underbrush and tall grass.
- If you are outdoors for a long time, check yourself several times during the day. Especially check in hairy areas of the body like the back of the neck and the scalp line.
- Inspect yourself carefully for insects or ticks after being out-doors or have someone else do it.
- Avoid walking in areas where snakes are known to live.
- If you encounter a snake, look around. There may be others. Turn around and walk away on the same path on which you came.
- Wear sturdy hiking boots.
- If you have pets that go outdoors, spray them with repellent made for that type of pet. Apply the repellent according to the label and check your pet for ticks often.
- If you will be in a grassy or wooded area for a long time, or if you know the area is highly infested with insects or ticks, consider using a repellent. Follow the directions carefully.

have rabies must get medical attention. Treatment for rabies includes a series of vaccine injections to build up immunity that will help fight the disease.

If someone is bitten by an animal, try to get him or her away from the animal without putting yourself in danger. Do not try to stop, hold or catch the animal.

To care for an animal bite—
- Control bleeding first if the wound is bleeding seriously.
- Do not clean serious wounds. The wound will be cleaned at a medical facility.
- Call 9-1-1 or the local emergency number if the wound is bleeding seriously or you suspect the animal might have rabies.
- Wash minor wounds with soap and water.
- Control any bleeding.

- Apply triple antibiotic ointment and a dressing.
- Watch for signals of infection.

If possible, try to remember what the animal looked like and the area in which you last saw it. When you call 9-1-1 or the local emergency number, the call taker will direct the proper authorities, such as animal control, to the scene.

Marine Life

The stings of some forms of marine life are not only painful, but they can actually make you sick (Fig. 10-7, A-D). The side effects include allergic reactions that can cause breathing and heart problems as well as paralysis. If you encounter someone who has a marine-life sting—
- Get a lifeguard to remove the person from the water as soon as possible. If a lifeguard is not available, use a reaching assist, if possible.
- Call 9-1-1 or the local emergency number if the person does not know what stung him or her, has a history of allergic reactions to marine-life stings, is stung on the face or neck or starts to have trouble breathing.
- If you know the sting is from a jellyfish, sea anemone or Portuguese man-of-war, soak the injured part in vinegar as soon as possible. Vinegar works best to offset the toxin, but rubbing alcohol or baking soda also may be used. Do not rub the wound or apply fresh water or ammonia because this increases pain.
- If you know the sting is from a stingray, sea urchin or spiny fish, flush the wound with tap water. Ocean water also may be used. Keep the injured part still and soak the affected area in non-scalding hot water (as hot as the person can stand) for about 30 minutes or until the pain goes away. If hot water is not available, packing the area in hot sand may have a similar effect if the sand is hot enough. Then carefully clean the wound and apply a bandage. Watch for signals of infection and check with a health-care provider to determine if a tetanus shot is needed.

Poisonous Plants

Every year, millions of people suffer from contact with poisonous plants such as poison ivy, poison oak and poison sumac (Fig. 10-8, A-C). You can often avoid or limit the irritating effects of touching or brushing against poisonous plans by following these steps:
- Remove exposed clothing and wash the exposed area thoroughly with soap and water as soon as possible after contact.

FIGURE 10-7, A-D The painful sting of some marine animals can cause serious problems: A, Stingray B, Portuguese man-of-war C, Sea anemone D, Jellyfish.

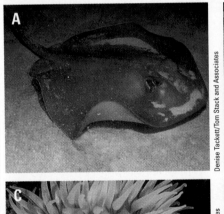
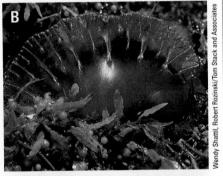
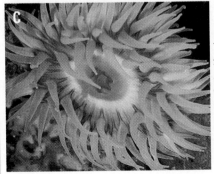
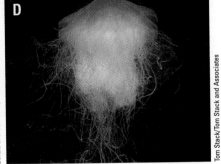

- Wash clothing exposed to plant oils since the oils can linger on fabric. Wash your hands thoroughly after handling exposed clothing. Wash your hands after touching exposed pets.

- Put a paste of baking soda and water on the area several times a day if a rash or weeping sore has already begun to develop. Calamine lotion and antihistamines, such as Benadryl®, may also help dry up the sores.

- See a health-care provider if the condition gets worse. The provider may decide to give anti-inflammatory drugs, such as corticosteroids or other medications, to relieve discomfort.

CRITICAL FACTS

CARING FOR BITES AND STINGS

Insect Bites
Signals
- Stinger may be present.
- Pain.
- Swelling.
- Possible allergic reaction.

Care
- Remove stinger—scrape it away or use tweezers.
- Wash wound.
- Cover.
- Apply a cold pack.
- Watch for signals of allergic reaction.

Spider Bite/Scorpion Sting
Signals
- Bite mark.
- Swelling.
- Pain.
- Nausea and vomiting.
- Trouble breathing or swallowing.

Care
- Wash wound.
- Apply a cold pack.
- Get medical care to receive antivenin.
- Call 9-1-1 or the local emergency number, if necessary.

Marine-Life Stings
Signals
- Possible marks.
- Pain.
- Swelling.
- Possible allergic reaction.

Care
- If jellyfish—soak area in vinegar.
- If stingray—soak area in nonscalding hot water until pain goes away. Clean and bandage wound.
- Call 9-1-1 or the local emergency number, if necessary.

Snake Bites
Signals
- Bite mark.
- Pain.

Care
Pit Vipers (Rattlesnake, Copperhead, Cottonmouth)
- Call 9-1-1 or the local emergency number.
- Wash wound.
- Keep bitten part still, and lower than the heart.

Elapid Snakes (Coral Snake)
- Call 9-1-1 or the local emergency number.
- Wash the wound.
- Keep bitten part still, and lower than the heart.
- Apply an elastic roller bandage.

Animal Bites
Signals
- Bite mark.
- Bleeding.

Care
- If bleeding is minor—wash wound.
- Control bleeding.
- Apply triple antibiotic ointment.
- Cover.
- Get medical attention if wound bleeds severely or if you suspect animal has rabies.
- Call local emergency number or contact animal control personnel.

FIGURE 10-8, A-C A, Poison ivy B, Poison sumac C, Poison oak.

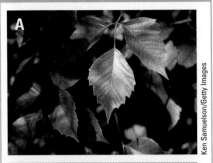

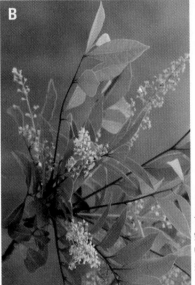

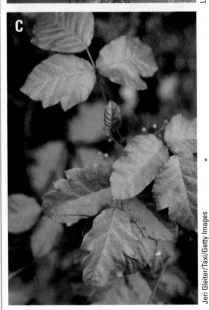

Ken Samuelson/Getty Images

Larry West/Taxi/Getty Images

Jeri Gleiter/Taxi/Getty Images

DID YOU KNOW?

HOW TO PREVENT POISONING

It only takes a moment for a small child to get into trouble. Children are curious and can get into things in ways you might not think possible. Almost all child poisonings take place when a child was being watched by a parent or guardian. Many substances found in or around the house are poisonous. Children are especially likely to be poisoned because they tend to put everything into their mouths.

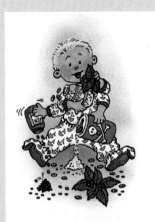

Follow these guidelines to guard against poisoning emergencies:

- Always supervise children closely, especially in areas where poisons are commonly stored, such as kitchens, bathrooms and garages.
- Keep all medications and household products locked away, well out of the reach of children.
- Install special clamps to keep children from opening cabinets.
- Consider all household or drugstore products to be potentially harmful.
- Use childproof safety caps on medicine containers and other potentially dangerous products.
- Never call medicine "candy" to get a child to take it, even if it has a pleasant candy flavor.
- Read all labels.
- Keep products in their original containers with the labels in place.
- Use poison symbols to identify dangerous substances and teach children what the symbols mean.
- Dispose of outdated products as recommended.
- Use chemicals only in well-ventilated areas.
- Set a good example during work or recreation that may put you in contact with a poisonous substance. Wear proper protective clothing, such as gloves, goggles or a mask.

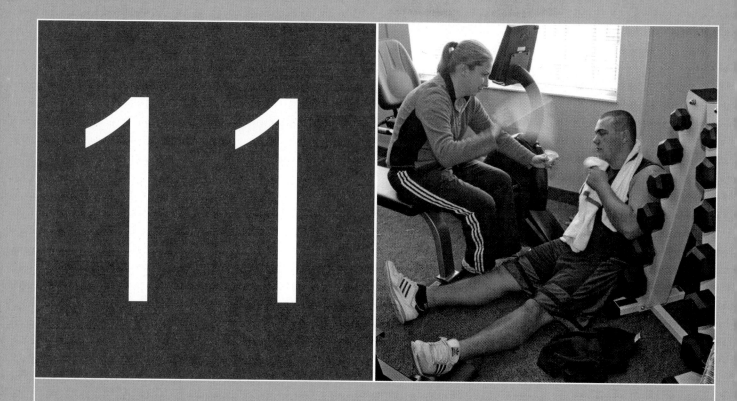

11

Once the signals of a heat- or cold-related emergency begin to appear, the person's condition can quickly become worse.

Chapter 11

Heat- or Cold-Related Emergencies

Exposure to extreme heat or cold can make a person seriously ill. The likelihood of illness also depends on factors such as physical activity, clothing, wind, humidity, working and living conditions and a person's age and state of mind (Fig. 11-1).

Once the signals of a heat- or cold-related illness begin to appear, a person's condition can quickly get worse. A heat- or cold-related emergency can result in death. If you see any of the signals of sudden illness and the person has been exposed to extremes of heat or cold, suspect a heat- or cold-related illness.

People at risk for heat- or cold-related emergencies include those who work or exercise outdoors, elderly people, young children and people with health problems. Also at risk are those who have had a heat- or cold-related illness in the past, those with medical conditions that cause poor blood circulation and those who take medications to get rid of water from the body (diuretics).

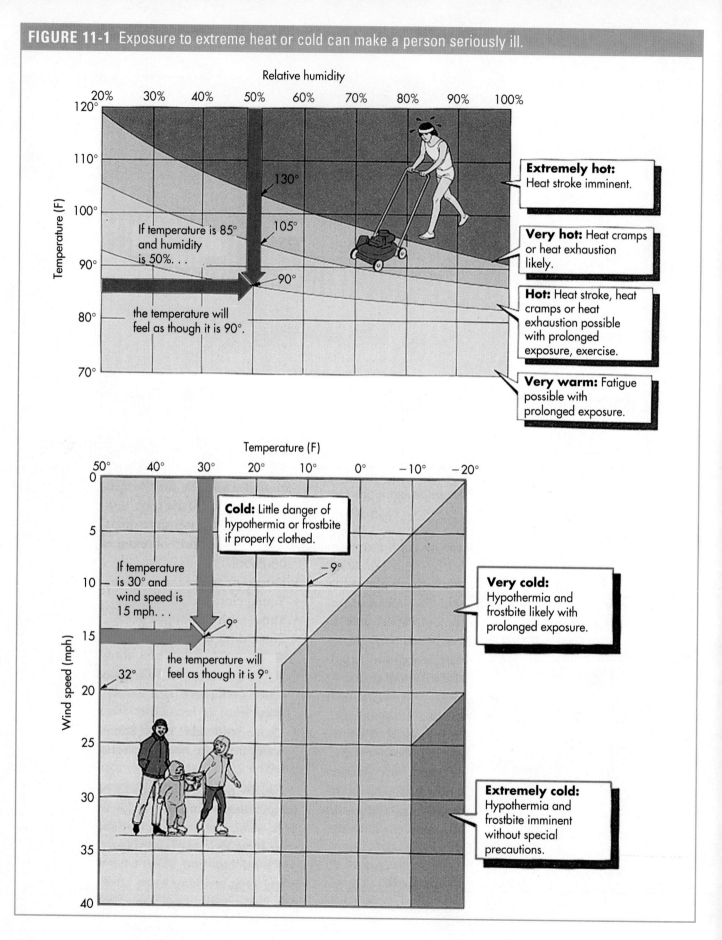

FIGURE 11-1 Exposure to extreme heat or cold can make a person seriously ill.

Relative humidity

Extremely hot: Heat stroke imminent.

Very hot: Heat cramps or heat exhaustion likely.

Hot: Heat stroke, heat cramps or heat exhaustion possible with prolonged exposure, exercise.

Very warm: Fatigue possible with prolonged exposure.

If temperature is 85° and humidity is 50%. . . the temperature will feel as though it is 90°.

Temperature (F)

Cold: Little danger of hypothermia or frostbite if properly clothed.

Very cold: Hypothermia and frostbite likely with prolonged exposure.

Extremely cold: Hypothermia and frostbite imminent without special precautions.

If temperature is 30° and wind speed is 15 mph. . . the temperature will feel as though it is 9°.

People usually try to get out of extreme heat or cold before they begin to feel ill. However, some people do not or cannot. Athletes and those who work outdoors often keep working even after they begin to feel ill. People living in buildings that are poorly ventilated, poorly insulated or with poor heating or cooling systems are at increased risk of heat- or cold-related emergencies. Often they might not even recognize they are in danger of becoming ill.

HEAT-RELATED ILLNESS

Heat cramps, heat exhaustion and heat stroke are conditions caused by overexposure to heat.

Heat Cramps

Heat cramps are the least severe and often are the first signals that the body is having trouble with the heat. Heat cramps are painful muscle spasms. They usually occur in the legs and abdomen. Think of them as a warning of a possible heat-related emergency.

Care for Heat Cramps. To care for heat cramps, have the person rest in a cool place. Give cool water or a commercial sports drink. Usually, rest and fluids are all the person will need to recover. Lightly stretch the muscle and gently massage the area (Fig. 11-2). The person should not take salt tablets or salt water. They can make the situation worse.

When cramps stop, the person can usually start activity again if there are no other signals of illness. He or she should keep drinking plenty of fluids. Watch the person carefully for further signals of heat-related illness.

Heat Exhaustion

Heat exhaustion is a more severe condition than heat cramps. It often affects athletes, firefighters, construction workers and factory workers, as well as those who wear heavy clothing in a hot, humid environment. Its signals

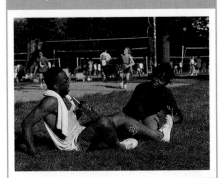

FIGURE 11-2 Lightly stretching the muscle and gently massaging the area, along with rest and fluids, is usually enough for the body to recover from heat cramps.

include cool, moist, pale, ashen or flushed skin; headache; nausea; dizziness; weakness; and exhaustion.

Heat Stroke

Heat stroke is the least common but most severe heat emergency. It most often occurs when people ignore the signals of heat exhaustion. Heat stroke develops when the body systems are overwhelmed by heat and begin to stop functioning. Heat stroke is a serious medical emergency. The signals of heat stroke include red skin that can be either dry or moist; changes in consciousness; rapid, weak pulse; and rapid, shallow breathing.

Care for Heat Exhaustion and Heat Stroke. When you recognize heat-related illness in its early stages, you can usually reverse it. Get the person out of the heat. Loosen any tight clothing and apply cool, wet cloths, such as towels or sheets, taking care to remoisten the cloths periodically (Fig. 11-3). Spraying the person with water and fanning is also beneficial. If the person is conscious, give him or her small amounts of cool water to drink.

SHADE
H2O

CARING FOR COLD-RELATED EMERGENCIES

Hypothermia

- Gently move the person to a warm place.
- Check ABCs and care for shock.
- Remove wet clothing and cover the person with blankets and plastic sheeting to hold in body heat.
- Carefully monitor use of heating pads and hot water bottles so that the person is not unintentionally burned.
- Warm the person slowly and handle the person carefully.

Frostbite

- Remove wet clothing and jewelry from the affected area.
- Soak the frostbitten area in warm water.
- Cover with dry, sterile dressings. Do not rub the frostbitten area.
- Check ABCs and care for shock.
- Do not rewarm a frostbitten part if there is a danger of it refreezing.

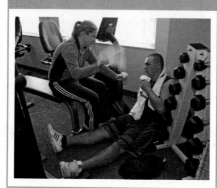

FIGURE 11-3 When you recognize a heat-related illness, get the person out of the heat, loosen any tight clothing and apply cool, wet cloths, such as towels or sheets.

Do not let the conscious person drink too quickly. Give about 4 ounces of water every 15 minutes. Let the person rest in a comfortable position and watch carefully for changes in his or her condition. The person should not resume normal activities the same day.

Refusing water, vomiting and changes in consciousness mean that the person's condition is getting worse. Call 9-1-1 or the local emergency number immediately if you have not already done so. If the person vomits, stop giving fluids and place the person on his or her side. Watch for signals of breathing problems. Keep the person lying down and continue to cool the body any way you can. If you have ice packs or cold packs, place them on each of the person's wrists and ankles, on the groin, in each armpit and on the neck to cool the large blood vessels. Use barriers, like towels or clothing, between the ice packs and the person to protect the skin. Do not apply rubbing (isopropyl) alcohol.

COLD-RELATED ILLNESS

Frostbite and hypothermia are two types of cold-related emergencies.

Frostbite

Frostbite is the freezing of body parts exposed to the cold. Severity depends on the air temperature, length of exposure and the wind. Frostbite can cause the loss of fingers, hands, arms, toes, feet and legs.

The signals of frostbite include lack of feeling in the affected area and skin that appears waxy, is cold to the touch or is discolored (flushed, white, yellow or blue).

Care for Frostbite. To care for frostbite, handle the area gently. Never rub an affected area. Rubbing causes further damage to soft tissues. Do not attempt to rewarm the frostbitten area if there is a chance that it might refreeze or if you are close to a medical facility. If you do warm the area, do so gently by soaking it in water not warmer than 105° F (Fig. 11-4, A). If you do not have a thermometer, test the water temperature yourself. If the temperature is uncomfortable to your touch, it is too warm. Keep the frostbitten part in the water until normal color returns and it feels warm. Loosely bandage the area with a dry, sterile dressing (Fig. 11-4, B). If fingers or toes are frostbitten, place cotton or gauze between them. Do not break any blisters. Take precautions to prevent hypothermia. Call 9-1-1 or seek emergency medical help as soon as possible.

Hypothermia

In a hypothermic condition, the entire body cools because its ability to keep warm fails. The person will die if not given care. Signals of hypothermia

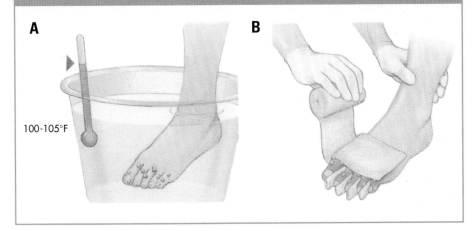

FIGURE 11-4, A-B A, To care for frostbite, warm the area gently by soaking the affected part in water not warmer than 105° F. Keep the frostbitten part in the water until normal color returns and it feels warm. B, Loosely bandage the area with a dry, sterile dressing.

A

100-105°F

B

include shivering, numbness, glassy stare, indifference and loss of consciousness. Shivering that stops without rewarming is a sign of deterioration and the need for immediate medical care.

The air temperature does not have to be below freezing for people to develop hypothermia, especially if the person is wet or if it is windy. Elderly people in poorly heated homes can

develop hypothermia at higher temperatures. The homeless, the ill and young children also are at risk. Substances that interfere with the body's normal response to cold, such as alcohol, may cause hypothermia to occur more easily. Any medical condition that impairs circulation, such as diabetes or cardiovascular disease, also can make a person more likely to develop hypothermia. Anyone remaining in cold

water or wet clothing for a long time may also easily develop hypothermia.

Care for Hypothermia. To care for hypothermia, start by caring for life-threatening conditions. Call 9-1-1 or the local emergency number. Make the person comfortable. Remove wet clothing and dry the person. Warm the body gradually by wrapping the person in blankets or putting on dry clothing and moving him or her to a warm place (Fig. 11-5). If they are available, apply heat pads or other heat sources to the body. Keep a barrier, such as a blanket, towel or clothing, between the heat source and the person to avoid burning him or her. If the person is alert, give warm liquids that do not contain alcohol or caffeine. Do not warm the person too quickly, such as by immersing the person in warm water. Rapid rewarming can cause dangerous heart problems. Handle the person gently.

Severe Hypothermia. In cases of severe hypothermia, the person may be unconscious. Breathing may have slowed or stopped. The pulse may be

The air temperature does not have to be below freezing for someone to develop hypothermia.

FIGURE 11-5 For hypothermia, warm the body gradually by wrapping the person in blankets or putting on dry clothing and moving him or her to a warm place.

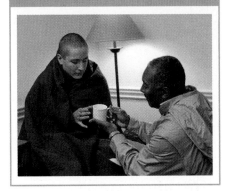

slow and irregular. In these circumstances, when checking for signs of life, the pulse should be checked for up to 30 to 45 seconds. The body may feel stiff because the muscles became rigid. Call 9-1-1 or the local emergency number. Keep checking breathing and signs of life. Give rescue breathing or cardiopulmonary resuscitation (CPR) if necessary. Continue to warm the person until emergency medical services (EMS) personnel arrive. Be prepared to start CPR and use an automated external defibrillator (AED), if appropriate.

PREVENTING HEAT- AND COLD-RELATED EMERGENCIES

In general, illnesses caused by overexposure to extreme temperatures can be prevented. To prevent heat- and cold-related emergencies, follow these guidelines:

- Avoid being outdoors in the hottest or coldest part of the day.
- Change your activity level according to the temperature.
- Take frequent breaks.
- Dress appropriately for the environment.
- Drink large amounts of fluids (Fig. 11-6).

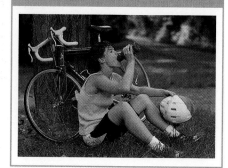

FIGURE 11-6 To avoid heat- and cold-related emergencies, take frequent breaks, dress appropriately for the environment and drink large amounts of fluids.

THE HIGH-TECH WAR AGAINST COLD

In the past, humans depended entirely on nature for clothing. Animal skins, furs and feathers protected us from freezing temperatures. As long as seasonal changes and cold climates exist, preventing cold-related illness, such as hypothermia, remains important when we work or play outside. Although natural fibers, such as wool and down, are still available, synthetic fibers now used in clothing make being outdoors in the cold a lot more comfortable.

The best way to use outdoor fabrics is to layer them. Layering creates warmth by trapping warm air between the layers to insulate the body. It enables you to regulate your body temperature and deal with changes in the environment. By wearing several layers of clothing, you can take clothes off when you become too warm and put them back on if you get cold.

Start off with an underwear layer. Commonly called long underwear, it includes thin, snug-fitting pants and a long-sleeved shirt. Underwear should supply you with basic insulation and pull moisture away from your skin. Damp, sweaty skin can chill you when you slow down or stop moving. Natural fibers, such as wool and silk, can be quite warm and are sufficient for light activity. For heavier exercise, however, synthetic fabrics absorb less moisture and actually carry water droplets away from your skin. Polypropylene™ and Capalene™ are two popular synthetic fabrics used for underwear.

Next, to provide additional warmth, add one or more insulating layers. The weight of insulating clothing should be considered in relation to planned activities, weather conditions and how efficiently the garment compresses to pack. Depending on the temperature, a wool sweater or a down jacket may provide an insulating layer for the upper body. But do not forget your legs. Wool pants are a better choice than jeans or corduroys. Synthetic materials used in jackets and pants include Thinsulate™, Quallofil™, Polartec™ and pile (a plush, nonpiling polyester fiber).

Although down is an excellent lightweight insulator, it becomes useless when wet, so a water-repellent or quick-drying fabric like pile may keep you warmer in a damp climate.

Finish with a windproof, and preferably waterproof, shell layer. Synthetic, high-tech fabrics make a strong showing here. Windproof fabrics have names like Supplex™, Silmond™, Captiva™ or ripstop nylon. Coatings, such as Hypalon™, applied to jackets and pants are completely water repellent. At the same time, most waterproof fabrics are "breathable." They repel wind and rain but allow perspiration to pass through the fabric so that you stay dry and warmer. Gore-Tex™, Thintech™, Ultrex™, and Super Microft™ are some of the names given to these fabrics. Pay close attention to vents and closures in garments. They should seal tightly and open freely to adapt to changing activities and weather conditions. It is also important to make sure your outer garments are big enough to fit over several layers of clothing.

A hat is vital to staying truly warm. Gloves, insulating socks, neck gaiters and headbands all protect you from the cold. Visit your local outdoor store for more information about the best clothing for your specific work or recreational activities.

SOURCES
National Ski Patrol, www.nsp.org/nsp2002/safety_info_template.asp?mode_dress. Accessed 10/29/04.
Recreation Equipment Incorporated: *Layering for comfort: FYI, an informational brochure from REI*, Seattle, 1991.
Recreation Equipment Incorporated: *Understanding outdoor fabrics: FYI, An informational brochure from REI*, Seattle, 1991.
Recreation Equipment Incorporated: *Outerwear product information guide*, Seattle, 1995.

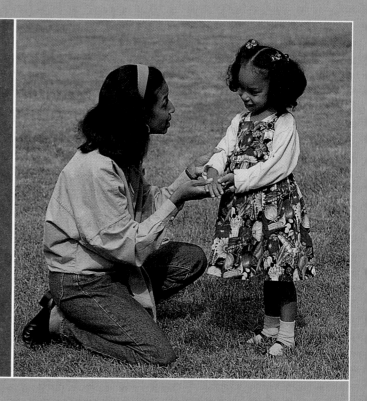

12

To help an ill or injured child, you will need to try to imagine how the child might feel.

Chapter 12

Special Situations and Circumstances

In an emergency, it is helpful to be aware of the special needs and considerations of children, older adults, people with disabilities and people who do not speak the same language you speak. It is also helpful to be prepared for other special circumstances including emergency childbirth and hostile situations. Knowing these needs and considerations will help you better understand the nature of the emergency and give appropriate care. A young child may be terrified. An elderly adult may be confused. A person with a disability may be unable to hear or see you. An immigrant may not speak English and you may not know his or her language. Being able to communicate with and reassure people with special needs will help you to care for them effectively.

INFANTS AND CHILDREN

Infants and children have unique needs and require special care. Assessing a conscious infant or child's condition can be difficult, especially if he or she does not know you. At certain ages, infants and children do not readily accept strangers. Infants and very young children cannot tell you what is wrong.

Communicating with an Ill or Injured Child

We tend to react more strongly and emotionally to a child who is in pain or terrified. In such a situation, you will need to try exceptionally hard to control your emotions and your facial expressions. Doing so will help both the child and concerned adults. To help an ill or injured child, you will also need to try to imagine how the child might feel. A child is afraid of the unknown. This includes being ill or hurt, touched by strangers and being separated from his or her parents or guardian.

How you interact with an ill or injured infant or child is very important. You need to reduce the child's anxiety and panic and gain the child's trust and cooperation, if possible. Move in slowly. The sudden appearance of a stranger may upset the child. Get as close to the infant's or child's eye level as you can, and keep your voice calm (Fig. 12-1). Smile at the child. Ask the child's name and use it when you talk with him or her. Talk slowly and distinctly, and use words the child will easily understand. Ask questions the child will be able to answer easily. Explain to the child and the parents or guardian what you are going to do. Reassure the child that you are there to help and will not leave him or her.

To be able to effectively check infants and children, it is helpful to be aware of certain characteristics of children in specific age groups.

Characteristics of Infants and Children

Children up to 1 year of age are commonly referred to as infants. Infants less than 6 months old are relatively easy to approach and are unlikely to be afraid of you. Older infants, however, often show "stranger anxiety."

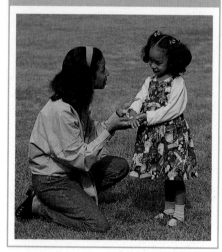

FIGURE 12-1 To communicate with a child, get as close to eye level as you can.

They may turn away from you and cry and cling to their parent or guardian. If a parent or the guardian is calm and cooperative, ask him or her to help you. Try to check the infant in the parent or guardian's lap or arms.

One- to 2-year-old children are commonly referred to as toddlers. Toddlers may not cooperate with your attempts to check them. They are usually concerned about being separated from a parent or guardian. If you reassure the toddler that he or she will not be separated from a parent or guardian, the toddler may be comforted. If possible, give the toddler a few minutes to get used to you before attempting to check him or her, and check the toddler in the parent or guardian's lap (Fig. 12-2, A). A toddler may also respond to praise or be comforted by holding a special toy or blanket.

Three- to 5-year-old children are commonly referred to as preschoolers. Children in this age group are usually easy to check if you make use of their natural curiosity. Allow them to inspect

items such as bandages. Opportunities to explore can reduce children's fears and distract them while you are checking them and giving care. Reassure the child that you are going to help and will not leave him or her. Sometimes you can show what you are going to do on a stuffed animal or doll (Fig. 12-2, B). The child may be upset by seeing his or her cut or other injury, so cover it with a dressing as soon as possible.

School-age children are between 6 and 12 years of age. They are usually cooperative and can be a good source of information about what happened. You can usually talk readily with school-age children. However, do not expect a child to always behave in a way consistent with his or her chronological age. An injured 11-year-old, for example, may behave more like a 7-year-old. Be especially careful not to talk down to these children. Let them know if you are going to do anything that may be painful. Children in this age group are becoming conscious of their bodies and may not like exposure. Respect their modesty.

Children between 13 and 18 years of age are considered adolescents. They typically behave more like adults than like children. Direct your questions to the adolescent rather than to a parent or guardian. Allow input from a parent or guardian, however. Occasionally, if a parent or guardian is present, you may not be able to get an accurate idea of what happened or what is wrong. Adolescents are modest and often react better to a responder of the same gender.

Interacting with Parents and Caregivers

If the family is excited or agitated, the child is likely to be, too. When you can calm the family, the child will often calm down as well. Remember to get consent to give care from any adult

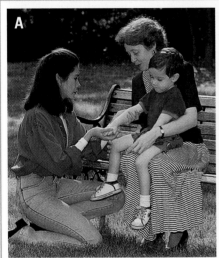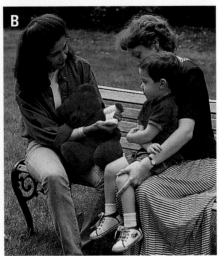

FIGURE 12-2, A-B A, Allow a parent to hold the child while you check him or her. B, Demonstrating first aid steps on a stuffed animal or doll helps a toddler understand how you will care for him or her.

responsible for the child when possible. Concerned adults need your support, so behave as calmly as possible. Remember to observe the whole situation and ask questions to see if there may be special needs to consider.

Some children and adults are dependent on technology, such as tracheotomy tubes, mechanical ventilators, feeding tubes or pacemakers. When caring for someone with special needs it is important to ask if they have an emergency information form summarizing vital information, including emergency contacts, names and phone numbers, allergies and other medical problems or issues.

Observing an Infant or Child

You can obtain a lot of information by observing the infant or child before actually touching him or her. Look for signals that indicate changes in the level of consciousness, trouble breathing and apparent injuries and conditions. Realize that the situation may change as soon as you touch the child

because he or she may become anxious or upset. Do not separate the infant or child from loved ones. Often a parent or guardian will be holding a crying infant or child. In this case, you can check the child while the adult continues to hold him or her. Unlike some ill or injured adults, an infant or child is unlikely to try to cover up or deny how he or she feels. An infant or child in pain, for example, will generally let you know that he or she hurts and will point out the source of the pain as well as he or she can.

Whenever possible, begin your check of a conscious child at the toe rather than the head. Checking this way is less threatening to the child and allows him or her to watch what is going on and take part in it. Ask a young child to point to any place that hurts. An older child can tell you the location of painful areas. If you need to hold an infant, always support the head when you pick him or her up. For more information on checking an infant or child, see Chapter 3.

Special Challenges

Certain problems are unique to children, such as specific kinds of injury and illness. The following sections discuss some of these concerns.

Injury. Injury is the number one cause of death for children in the United States. Many of these deaths are the result of motor vehicle crashes. The greatest dangers to a child involved in a motor vehicle incident are airway obstruction and bleeding. Severe bleeding must be controlled as quickly as possible. A relatively small amount of blood lost by an adult is a large amount for an infant or child. Because a child's head is large and heavy in proportion to the rest of the body, the head is the most often injured area. A child injured as the result of force or a blow may also have damage to the organs in the abdominal and chest cavities. Such damage can cause severe internal bleeding. A child secured only by a lap belt may have serious abdominal or spinal injuries in a car crash. Try to find out what happened, because a severely injured child may not immediately show signals of injury.

To avoid needless deaths of children caused by motor vehicle crashes, laws have been enacted requiring that children ride in safety seats or wear safety belts. As a result, more children's lives are saved. You may have to check and care for an injured child while he or she is in a safety seat. A safety seat does not normally pose problems while you are checking a child. Leave the child in the seat if the seat has not been damaged. If the child is to be transported to a medical facility for examination, he or she can often be safely secured in the safety seat for transport.

Illness. Certain signals in an infant or child can indicate specific illnesses. These illnesses usually are not life threatening, but some can be. A high fever in a child often indicates some form of infection. In a young child, even a minor infection can result in a rather high fever—usually defined as a temperature above 103° F (40° C). Prolonged or excessively high fever can result in seizures.

Your initial care for a child with a high fever is to gently cool the child. Remove excessive clothing or blankets and sponge the child with lukewarm water. Call a physician immediately. *Do not give the child aspirin.* For a child, taking aspirin can result in an extremely serious medical condition called *Reye's syndrome.* See Chapter 4 for details on breathing emergencies in infants and children.

Poisoning. Poisoning is the fifth-leading cause of unintentional death in the United States for people ages 1 to 24. For the youngest of these victims, mainly children under 5 years of age, poisoning often occurs from ingesting household products or medications. How to prevent and care for poisoning is discussed in Chapter 10.

Child Abuse. At some point, you may encounter a situation involving an injured child in which you have reason to suspect child abuse. *Child abuse* is the physical, psychological or sexual assault of a child resulting in injury and emotional trauma. Child abuse involves an injury or a pattern of injuries that do not result from an accident. Suspect child abuse if the child's injuries cannot be logically explained, or if a parent or guardian gives an inconsistent or suspicious account of how the injuries occurred.

The signals of child abuse include—
- An injury whose cause does not fit the parent or guardian's explanation.
- Obvious or suspected fractures in a child younger than 2 years of age.

- Any unexplained fractures.
- Injuries in various stages of healing, especially bruises and burns.
- Bruises and burns in unusual shapes, such as bruises shaped like belt buckles or burns the size of a cigarette tip.
- Unexplained lacerations or abrasions, especially to the mouth, lips and eyes.
- Injuries to the genitalia.
- Pain when the child sits down.
- More injuries than are common for a child of the same age.

When caring for a child who may have been abused, your first priority is to care for the child's illness or injuries. An abused child may be frightened, hysterical or withdrawn. He or she may be unwilling to talk about the incident in an attempt to protect the abuser. If you suspect abuse, explain your concerns to responding police officers or emergency medical services (EMS) personnel if possible.

If you think you have reasonable cause to believe that abuse has occurred, report your suspicions to a community or state agency, such as the Department of Social Services, the Department of Child and Family Services or Child Protective Services. You may be afraid to report suspected child abuse because you do not wish to get involved or are afraid of getting sued. However, in most states, when you make a report in good faith, you are immune from any civil or criminal liability or penalty, even if you made a mistake. In this instance, "good faith" means that you honestly believe that abuse has occurred or the potential for abuse exists and a prudent and reasonable person in the same position would also honestly believe abuse has occurred or the potential for abuse exists. You do not need to identify yourself when you report child

abuse, although your report will have more credibility if you do.

Sudden Infant Death Syndrome. *Sudden infant death syndrome (SIDS)* is a disorder that causes seemingly healthy infants to stop breathing while they sleep. SIDS is a leading cause of death for infants between 1 month and 1 year of age. By the time the infant's condition has been discovered, he or she will be in cardiac arrest. If you encounter an infant in this condition, make sure someone has called 9-1-1 or the local emergency number or call yourself. Perform cardiopulmonary resuscitation (CPR) on the infant until EMS personnel arrive.

An incident involving a severely injured or ill infant or child or one who has died can be emotionally upsetting. After such an episode, find someone you trust with whom you can talk about the experience and express your feelings. If you continue to be distressed, seek some professional counseling. The feelings caused by such incidents need to be dealt with and understood or they can result in serious stress reactions.

OLDER ADULTS

Older adults, or the elderly, are generally considered those people over 65 years of age. They are quickly becoming the fastest-growing age group in the United States. Since 1900, life expectancy in the United States has increased by 57 percent. In 1900, for example, the average life expectancy was 49 years. Today, it is over 75 years. The main explanations for the increase in life expectancy are medical advancements and improvements in health care.

Normal aging brings about changes. People age at different rates, however, and so do their organs and body parts. A person may have a "young" heart but "old" skin, for example, and someone with wrinkled, fragile skin may have strong bones or excellent respiratory function.

Overall, however, body function generally declines as we age, with some changes beginning as early as age 30. The lungs become less efficient, so older people are at higher risk of developing pneumonia and other lung diseases. The amount of blood pumped by the heart with each beat decreases, and the heart rate slows. The blood vessels harden, causing increased work for the heart. Hearing and vision usually decline, often causing some degree of sight and hearing loss. Reflexes become slower, and arthritis may affect joints, causing movement to become painful. Four out of five older adults develop some sort of chronic condition or disease.

Checking an Older Adult

Physical and mental changes can occur as a result of aging. Because of these changes, many older adults are particularly susceptible to certain problems. These problems may require you to adapt your way of communicating and to be aware of certain potential age-related conditions.

To check an injured or ill older adult, attempt to learn the person's name and use it when you speak to him or her. Consider using "Mrs.," "Mr." or "Ms." as a sign of respect. Make sure you are at the person's eye level so that he or she can see and hear you more clearly (Fig. 12-3). If the person seems confused at first, the confusion may be the result of impaired vision or hearing. If he or she usually wears eyeglasses and cannot find them, try to locate them. Speak slowly and clearly, and look at the person's face while you talk. Notice if he or she has a hearing aid. Someone who needs glasses to see or a hearing aid to hear is likely to be very anxious

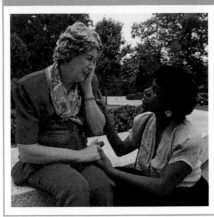

FIGURE 12-3 Speak to an elderly person at eye level so that he or she can see or hear you more clearly.

without them. If the person is truly confused, try to find out if the confusion is the result of the injury or an existing condition. Be sure to get as much information as possible from family members or bystanders. The person may be afraid of falling, so if he or she is standing, offer an arm or hand. Remember that an older person may need to move very slowly.

Try to find out what medications the person is taking so that you can tell EMS personnel. Look for a medical ID tag that will list the person's name, address and medical information. Be aware that an elderly person may not recognize the signals of a serious condition. An elderly person may also minimize any signals for fear of losing his or her independence or being placed in a nursing home.

Falls. Falls are the sixth-leading cause of death for people over 65 years of age. As a result of slower reflexes, failing eyesight and hearing, arthritis and problems such as unsteady balance and movement, older adults are at increased risk of falls. Falls fre-

quently result in fractures because the bones become weaker and more brittle with age.

Head Injuries. An older adult also is at greater risk of serious head injuries. As we age, the size of the brain decreases. This decrease results in more space between the surface of the brain and the inside of the skull. This space allows more movement of the brain within the skull, which can increase the likelihood of serious head injury. Occasionally, an older adult may not develop the signals of a head injury until days after a fall. Therefore, unless you know the cause of a behavior change, you should always suspect a head injury as a possible cause of unusual behavior in an elderly person, especially if the victim has had a fall or a blow to the head.

Confusion. The elderly are at increased risk of altered thinking patterns and confusion. Some of this change is the result of aging. Certain diseases, such as Alzheimer's disease, affect the brain, resulting in impaired memory and thinking and altered behavior. Confusion that comes on suddenly, however, may be the result of medication, even a medication the person has been taking regularly. An ill or injured person who has problems seeing or hearing may also become confused when ill or injured. This problem increases when the person is in an unfamiliar environment. A head injury can also result in confusion.

Confusion can be a signal of a medical emergency. An elderly person with pneumonia, for example, may not run a fever, have chest pain or be coughing, but because not enough oxygen is reaching the brain, the person may be confused. An elderly person can have a serious infection without fever, pain or nausea. An elderly person having a heart attack may not have chest pain, pale or ashen skin or other classic signals, but may be restless, short of breath and confused.

Depression is common in older adults. A depressed older adult may seem confused at first. A depressed person may also have signals, such as sudden shortness of breath or chest pains, with no apparent cause. Whatever the reason for any confusion, do not talk down to the elderly person or treat him or her like a child.

Problems with Heat and Cold. An elderly person is more susceptible to extremes in temperature. The person may be unable to feel temperature extremes because his or her body may no longer regulate temperature effectively. Body temperature may change rapidly to a dangerously high or low level.

The body of an elderly person retains heat because of a decreased ability to sweat and the reduced ability of the circulatory system to adjust to heat. If an elderly person shows signals of heat-related illness, take his or her temperature, and if it is above normal, call 9-1-1 or the local emergency number. Slowly cool the person off with a lukewarm sponge bath, and give care as described in Chapter 11. If you find an elderly person hot to the touch, unable to speak and unconscious or semiconscious, call 9-1-1 or the local emergency number immediately. Put the person in a cooler location if possible, but do not try to quickly cool the person with cold water or put him or her in front of a fan or air conditioner.

An elderly person may become chilled and suffer hypothermia simply by sitting in a draft or in front of a fan or air conditioner. Hypothermia can occur at any time of the year in temperature that is 65° F (18° C) or less. People can go on for several days suffering from mild hypothermia that they do not recognize. The older person with mild hypothermia will want to lie down frequently, which will lower the body temperature even further. If you suspect hypothermia, feel the person's skin to see if it is cold. Take the person's temperature. If his or her temperature is below 98.6° F (37° C)—

- Put the person in a warm room.
- Wrap him or her in one or two blankets.
- Give the person warm, decaffeinated and non-alcoholic liquid to drink.
- Call a physician for advice.

However, if the body temperature is below 95° F (35° C), call 9-1-1 or the local emergency number immediately. This condition is life threatening. Do not apply direct heat, such as a heating pad, electric blanket turned to high or a hot bath. Doing so will cause blood flow to increase to the area being heated and take blood away from the vital organs.

EMERGENCY CHILDBIRTH

Words such as exhausting, stressful, exciting, fulfilling, painful and scary are sometimes used to describe a planned childbirth: one that occurs in the hospital or at home under the supervision of a health-care provider. If you find yourself assisting with the delivery of a newborn, however, it will probably not be happening in a planned situation. Therefore, your feelings, as well as those of the expectant mother, may be intensified by fear of the unexpected or the possibility that something might go wrong.

Take comfort in knowing that things rarely go wrong. Childbirth is a natural process. Thousands of children all over the world are born each day, without complications, in areas where no medical care is available.

By following a few simple steps, you can effectively assist in the birth process. If a woman is giving birth—

- Call 9-1-1 or the local emergency number.
- Give the EMS call taker the following important information:
  - The woman's name, age, and expected due date
  - How long she has been having labor pains
  - If this is her first child
- Talk with the woman to help her remain calm.
- Place layers of newspaper covered with layers of linens, towels or blankets under her.
- Control the scene so that the woman will have privacy.
- Position the woman on her back with her knees bent, feet flat and legs spread wide apart.
- Remember, the woman delivers the baby, so be patient and let it happen naturally.
- The baby will be slippery; avoid dropping the baby.
- Keep the baby warm.

CAUTIONS—

- Do not let the woman get up or leave to find a bathroom (most women have a desire to use the restroom).
- Do not hold her knees together; this will not slow the birth process and may complicate the birth or harm the baby.
- Do not place your fingers in the vagina for any reason.
- Do not pull on the baby.

PEOPLE WITH DISABILITIES

The absence or loss of motor, sensory or mental ability is called a *disability*. If a particular ability or function is damaged or reduced, it is considered to be impaired. People who have a disability may be impaired in one or more functions. The Centers for Disease Control and Prevention (CDC) estimates that over 33 million people in the United States have disabilities.

With many disabled people, communication can be a major challenge in finding out what has happened and what might be wrong in an emergency situation.

Physical Disability

A person is considered physically disabled if his or her ability to move (also called *motor function*) is impaired. A person is also considered physically disabled if his or her sensory function is impaired. Sensory function includes all of the senses—sight, hearing, taste, smell and touch. A person can be disabled in motor functions, sensory functions or both.

General hints for approaching an injured or ill person who you have reason to believe is disabled include—

- Speak to the person before touching him or her.
- Ask "How can I help?" or "Do you need help?"
- Ask for assistance and information from the person who has the disability—he or she has been living with the disability and best understands it. If the person is not able to communicate, ask family members, friends or companions who are available.
- Do not remove any braces, canes, other physical support, eyeglasses or hearing aids. Removal of these items may take away necessary physical support for the person's body.
- Look for a medical ID tag or bracelet at the person's wrist or neck.
- A person with a disability may have an animal assistant, such as a guide or hearing dog. Be aware that this animal may be protective of the person in an emergency situation. Someone may need to calm and restrain the animal. Allow the animal to stay with the person if possible, which will help reassure them both.

Hearing Loss

Hearing loss is defined as a partial or total loss of hearing. Some people are born with a hearing loss. Hearing loss can also result from an injury or illness affecting the ear, the nerves leading from the brain to the ear or the brain itself. You may not immediately realize that the injured or ill person has a hearing loss. Often the victim will tell you, either in speech or by pointing to the ear and shaking the head no. Some people carry a card stating that they have a hearing loss. You may see a hearing aid in a person's ear.

The biggest obstacle you must overcome in caring for a person with a hearing loss is communication. You will need to figure out how to get that person's consent to give care, and you will need to assess the problem.

Often the injured or ill person will be able to read lips. To assist him or her, position yourself where the person can clearly see your face. Look straight at the person while you speak, and speak slowly. Do not exaggerate the way you form words. Do not turn your face away while you speak. Many people with a hearing impairment, however, do not read lips. In these cases, using gestures and writing messages on paper may be the most effective way to communicate.

If you and the victim know sign language, use it. Some people who are hearing impaired have a machine called a telecommunications device for the deaf (TDD). You can use this device to type messages and questions to the victim, and the victim can type replies to you (Fig. 12-4, A-D).

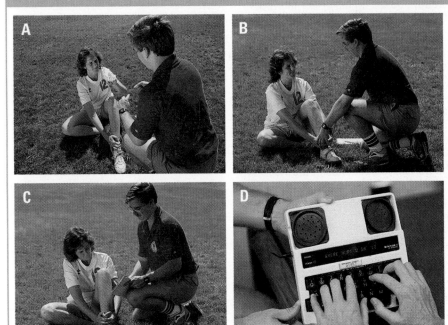

FIGURE 12-4, A-D Communicate with a person who has a hearing loss in the best way possible: A, Using sign language, B, lip reading, C, writing or D, using a telecommunications device for the deaf.

Many people who have a hearing impairment can speak, some distinctly, some not so clearly. If you have trouble understanding, ask the person to repeat what he or she said. Do not pretend to understand.

Vision Loss

Vision loss is a partial or total loss of sight. Vision loss can have many causes. Some people are born with vision loss. Others lose vision as a result of disease or injury. Vision loss is not necessarily a problem with the eyes. It can result from problems with the vision centers in the brain.

People with vision loss are generally not embarrassed by their condition. It is no more difficult to communicate orally with a person who has a partial or total loss of sight than with someone who can see. You do not need to speak loudly or in overly simple terms. Checking a person who has a vision loss is like checking a victim who has normal vision. The victim may not be able to tell you certain things about how an injury occurred, but can usually give you a generally accurate account based on his or her interpretation of sound and touch.

When caring for a person with vision loss, help to reassure him or her by explaining what is going on and what you are doing. If you must move a visually impaired person who can walk, stand beside the person and have him or her hold onto your arm (Fig.12-5). Walk at a normal pace, alert the person to obstacles in the way, such as stairs, and let the person know whether to step up or down. If the person has a seeing-eye dog, try to keep them together. Ask the person to tell you how to handle the dog or ask him or her to do it.

Motor Impairment

A person with motor impairment is unable to move normally. He or she may be missing a body part or have a

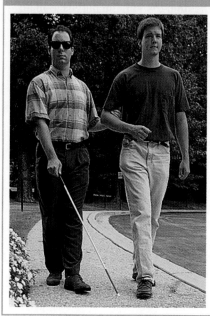

FIGURE 12-5 If a person with a vision loss can walk, stand beside him or her and have the person hold your arm.

problem with the bones or muscles or the nerves that control movement. Causes of motor impairment include stroke, muscular dystrophy, multiple sclerosis, paralysis, cerebral palsy or loss of a limb. When caring for an injured or ill person with motor impairment, be aware that the person may view accepting help as failure and may refuse your help to prove that he or she does not need it.

Determining which problems are preexisting and which are the result of immediate injury or illness can be difficult. If you care for all problems you detect as if they are new, you can hardly go wrong. Be aware that checking one side of the body against the other in your check for nonlife-threatening conditions may not be effective with a person with motor impairment, since body parts may not look normal.

Mental Impairment

Mental, or cognitive, function includes the brain's capacity to reason and process information. A person with mental impairment has problems performing these operations. Some types of mental impairment are genetic. Others result from injuries or infections that occur during pregnancy, shortly after birth or later in life. Some causes are never determined.

In some situations you will not be able to determine if a victim is mentally impaired; in others, it will be obvious. If you suspect that a person is mentally impaired, approach him or her as you would any other person in his or her age group. If the person appears not to understand you, rephrase what you were saying in simpler terms. Listen carefully to what the person says. People who are mentally impaired often lead very orderly and structured lives. A sudden illness or injury can disrupt this order and cause a great deal of anxiety and fear. Take time to explain who you are and what you are going to do. Offer reassurance. Try to gain the victim's trust. If a parent, guardian or caregiver is present, ask that person to help you care for the person.

People with certain types of mental illness might misinterpret your actions as being hostile or might be experiencing a different type of reality and may not understand you. You might need to act as if you are a part of that reality or you might need to back off and call 9-1-1 or the local emergency number, explaining that you think there is a psychiatric emergency. As you wait for professional help, try to keep track of where the person is and what he or she is doing so you can report it.

LANGUAGE BARRIERS

Another reason for an uncertain look when you speak to a victim is that the person may not understand English or any other language you may speak. Getting consent to give care to a victim with whom you have a language barrier can be a problem. Find out if any bystanders speak the victim's language and can help translate. Do your best to communicate non-verbally. Use gestures and facial expressions. If the person is in pain, he or she will probably be anxious to let you know where that pain is. Watch his or her gestures and facial expressions carefully.

When you speak to the victim, speak slowly and in a normal tone. The victim probably will have no trouble hearing you. When you call 9-1-1 or the local emergency number, explain that you are having difficulty communicating with the victim and say what nationality you believe the victim is or the language you believe the victim speaks. The EMS system may have someone available who can help with communication. If the victim has a life-threatening condition, such as severe bleeding, consent is implied.

CRIME SCENES AND HOSTILE SITUATIONS

In certain situations, such as a crime scene or an injured person who is hostile, you will need to use extreme caution. Although your first reaction may be to go to the aid of a victim, in these situations you should call 9-1-1 or the local emergency number and stay at a safe distance until the scene is secured.

Do not enter the scene of a suicide. If you happen to be on the scene when an unarmed person threatens suicide, call 9-1-1 or the local emergency number and the police. If the scene is safe, listen to the person and try to keep him or her talking until help arrives. Do not argue with the person. Leave or do not enter any scene where there is a weapon or where a crime has been committed. Do not approach the scene of a physical or sexual assault. These are crime scenes. Call 9-1-1 or the local emergency number and stay at a safe distance.

Sometimes a victim may be hostile or angry. A victim's rage or hostility may be caused by the injury, pain or fear. Some victims, afraid of losing control, will act resentful and suspicious. Hostile behavior may also result from the use of alcohol or other drugs, lack of oxygen or a medical condition. Once a victim realizes that you are there to help and are not a threat, the hostility usually goes away. If a victim refuses your care or threatens you, withdraw. Never try to argue with or restrain a victim. Call 9-1-1 or the local emergency number if someone has not already done so.

Uninjured family members may also display anger. They may pressure you to do something immediately. Often this anger stems from panic, anxiety or guilt. Try to remain calm, and be sympathetic but firm. Explain what you are going to do. If possible, find a way that family members can help, such as by comforting the victim.

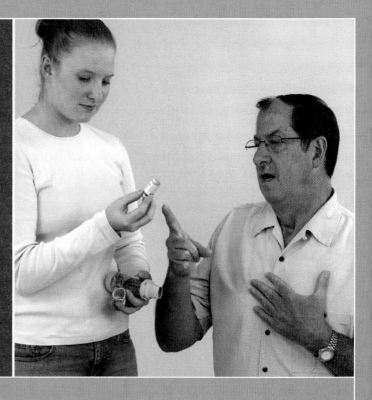

13

Severe asthma and deaths from asthma are increasing. It is likely that first aid responders may be asked to help people with breathing emergencies caused by asthma.

Chapter 13

Asthma

The instructions in this chapter are not a substitute for the directions that a medical professional gives to a person or gives as a consultation for a site where this equipment will be used. Consult a health-care professional for specific advice on use of this equipment.

ASTHMA

Asthma is an ongoing illness in which airways (small tubes in the lungs through which we breathe) have ongoing swelling. An asthma attack happens when a trigger, such as exercise, cold air, allergens or other irritants, affects the airways causing them to suddenly swell and narrow. This makes breathing difficult, which can be frightening (Fig. 13-1).

The Centers for Disease Control and Prevention (CDC) estimates that in 2003, nearly 30 million Americans were affected by asthma. Asthma is more common in children and young adults than in older adults, but its frequency and severity is increasing in all age groups in the United States. Asthma is the third-ranking cause of hospitalization among those younger than age 15.

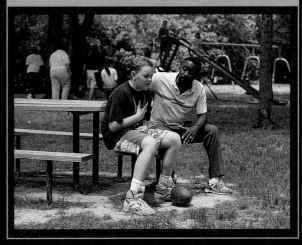

FIGURE 13-1 A person who is having trouble breathing may breathe more easily in a sitting position.

You can often tell when a person is having an asthma attack by the hoarse whistling sound he or she makes while exhaling. This sound, known as wheezing, occurs because air becomes trapped in the lungs. Coughing after exercise, crying or laughing are other signals that an asthma attack is taking place. Usually, people diagnosed with asthma control their attacks by controlling environmental variables and through medication and other forms of treatment. The medications stop the muscle spasm and open the airway, which makes breathing easier. Controlling the environmental variables, whenever possible, helps to reduce the triggers that can lead to the start of an asthma attack.

Triggers

A trigger is anything that sets off or starts an asthma attack. A trigger for one person is not necessarily a trigger for another. Some asthma triggers are—

- Dust, smoke and air pollution.
- Fear or anxiety.
- Hard exercise.
- Plants and molds.
- Perfume.
- Colds.
- Medications, such as aspirin.
- Animal fur or feathers.
- Temperature extremes and changes in the weather.

These are only a few of the things that can trigger asthma in some people.

Limiting Triggers in the Home. You can reduce the chances of triggering an asthma attack at home by—

- Keeping plants outside.
- Washing bedclothes weekly in hot water.
- Using hypoallergenic covers on mattresses and pillows.
- Eliminating or reducing the number of carpets and rugs.
- Regularly steam cleaning all carpets, rugs and upholstery.

- Keeping the home clean and free of dust and pests—wet dusting can be more effective than dry dusting.
- Not allowing, or being around, smoking.
- Changing the air filter in the central air or heating unit regularly.
- Eliminating or minimizing the number of stuffed toys.
- Using hypoallergenic health and beauty products.
- Washing pets weekly.
- Keeping pets outside of the house.

Emotions. Certain strong emotions can trigger an asthma attack. When a person feels a strong emotion, such as anger or fear, the following suggestions can reduce the chances that the emotions will trigger an asthma attack:

- Take a long deep breath in through the nose and slowly let it out through the mouth.
- Count to 10.
- Talk with a family member, trusted friend or health-care provider.
- Do a relaxing activity.

Infections. Colds and other respiratory infections can make an asthma condition worse. One of the most common ways people catch colds is by rubbing their noses or eyes with hands contaminated with a cold virus. Contamination often occurs by touching surfaces (such as doorknobs) or objects that other people have touched.

Some ways to reduce the chances of getting a cold or other respiratory infection [NOTE: these steps will not prevent human immunodeficiency virus (HIV), hepatitis, or some other viral infections] include—

- Washing hands regularly, especially after using the restroom, shaking hands with other people and before eating.
  - Effective handwashing, according to the CDC includes—
    - Wetting the hands and applying liquid or clean bar soap.

- Placing the bar soap on a rack and allowing it to drain.
- Rubbing the hands vigorously together and scrubbing all surfaces for at least 15 seconds or about the length of a little tune. It is the soap combined with the scrubbing action that helps dislodge and remove germs.
- Rinsing well and drying the hands.
- Cleaning environmental surfaces, such as telephones and counters, with a virus-killing disinfectant. The viruses that cause colds can survive up to 3 hours on objects such as telephones, counters and stair railings, so disinfecting them regularly might help prevent the spread of colds and viruses.
- Getting vaccinated for illnesses that have a vaccine available, such as influenza and whooping cough (pertussis).

Your health-care provider might have other suggestions based on your medical history.

Environment. Sudden changes in the weather, heavy mold or pollen content in the air and pollution all can trigger an asthma attack. To avoid attacks brought on by environmental triggers, people with asthma can—

- Wear the right clothing for the weather conditions.
- Stay indoors on days when there are significantly high risks of respiratory difficulties.
- Take preventative medications, as prescribed by a health-care provider.
- Avoid places with high amounts of dirt, smoke and other irritants.
- Notice how the weather affects their conditions and talk to their health-care provider about other prevention strategies.

Exercise. Exercise-induced asthma occurs during or shortly following intense exercise. Having this type of asthma does not mean a person cannot or should not exercise or play sports. A person should, however, recognize that he or she has exercise-induced asthma and do the following:

- Take prescribed medications 30 to 60 minutes before exercising.
- Slowly warm up prior to exercising, and cool down gently after exercising.
- Ensure proper hydration during exercise.
- Seek and follow the advice of his or her health-care provider.
- If participating in organized sports, notify his or her coach of the person's condition.

Medications

Some anti-inflammatory medications prescribed for the long-term control of asthma are taken daily (Fig. 13-2). Other medications are prescribed for quick relief and are taken only when a person is experiencing the signals of an asthma attack (Fig. 13-3). These medications help relieve the sudden swelling and are called *bronchodilators*.

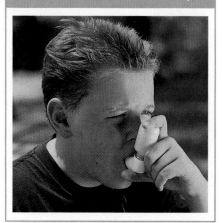

FIGURE 13-2 Some anti-inflammatory medications prescribed for the long-term control of asthma are taken daily.

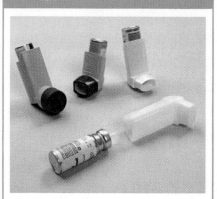

FIGURE 13-3 Some asthma medications are prescribed for quick relief and are taken only when a person is experiencing the signals of an asthma attack.

Signals of an Asthma Attack

- Coughing or wheezing noises
- Difficulty breathing, shortness of breath
- Rapid, shallow breathing
- Sweating
- Tightness in the chest
- Inability to talk without stopping for breath
- Feeling of fear or confusion

Assisting with Asthma Inhaler

Remember: Always obtain consent and wash your hands immediately after giving care.

To care for the person—

STEP 1
Help the person sit up and rest in a position comfortable for breathing.

STEP 2
If the person has medication for asthma, help him or her take it.

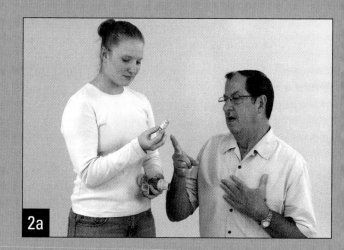

- **Ensure that the prescription is in the person's name and is prescribed for "quick relief"** or "acute" attacks. (NOTE: some inhalers contain long-acting, preventive medication that should NOT be used in the event of an emergency.)
- **Ensure that the expiration date of the medication has not passed.**
- **Read and follow all instructions** printed on the inhaler prior to administering the medication to the person.
- **Shake the inhaler.**
- **Remove the cover** from the inhaler mouthpiece. (Some inhalers have extension or spacer tubes that fit between the mouthpiece and the medication canister. If present, attach and use.)
- **Tell the person to breathe out as much as possible.**
- **Have the person place his or her lips tightly around the mouthpiece.** (NOTE: the person may use different techniques.)

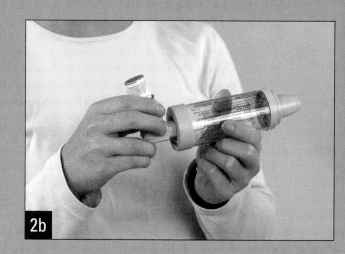

- As the person breathes in slowly, **administer the medication by quickly pressing down on the inhaler canister,** or the person may self-administer the medication—
  - The person should continue a full, deep breath.
  - Tell the person to try to hold his or her breath for a count of 10.
    - When using an extension tube have the person take 5 to 6 deep breaths through the tube without holding his or her breath.
- **Note the time of administration and any change in the person's condition.**
- The medication may be repeated once after 1 to 2 minutes.
  - NOTE: The medication may be repeated every 5 to 10 minutes thereafter, as needed, for areas with long EMS response times such as rural locations.
  - These medications might take 5 to 15 minutes to reach full effectiveness.

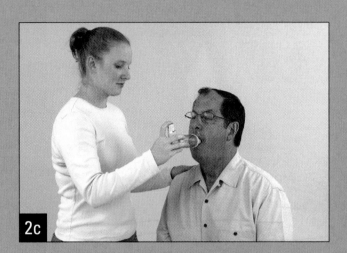

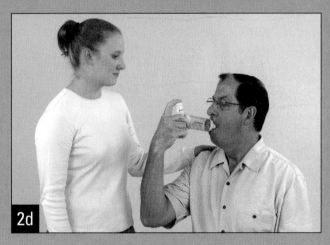

STEP 3
Stay with the person and monitor his or her condition and give care for any other injuries. Have the person rinse his or her mouth out with water.

STEP 4
Care for shock. Keep the person from getting chilled or overheated.
Check the scene and the person.
Call 9-1-1 or the local emergency number if trouble breathing does not improve quickly.

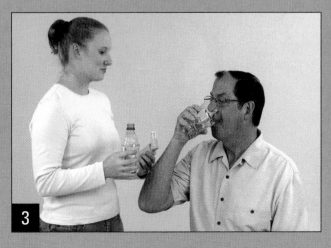

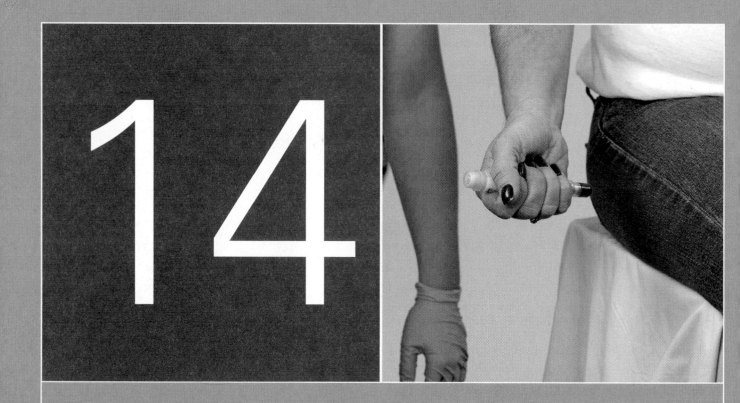

14

Allergic reactions are caused by the activity of the immune system.

Chapter 14

Anaphylaxis and Epinephrine Auto-Injectors

The instructions in this chapter are not a substitute for the directions that a medical professional gives to a person or gives as a consultation for a site where this equipment will be used. Consult a health-care professional for specific advice on use of this equipment.

ANAPHYLAXIS

Every year in the United States, between 400 and 800 deaths are caused by severe allergic reactions. These reactions bring on a condition called *anaphylactic shock,* also known as *anaphylaxis.*

A person can die from anaphylaxis within just 1 minute of being exposed to an *antigen*—a foreign substance that brings on the allergic reaction. Fortunately, some deaths can be prevented if anaphylaxis is recognized early and cared for quickly.

Allergic Reactions

Allergic reactions are caused by the activity of the immune system. The body recognizes and protects itself from antigens (foreign substances) by producing *antibodies,* which fight antigens. Antibodies are found in the liver, bone marrow, spleen and lymph glands. The *immune system* recognizes the antigens and releases chemicals to fight these foreign substances and eliminate them from the body.

These reactions range from mild to very severe: for instance, the common mild reaction to poison ivy (skin irritation) to a life-threatening reaction (swelling of the airway, trouble breathing and obstructed airway).

Some common antigens include but may not be limited to bee or insect venom, antibiotics, pollen, animal dander, sulfa, and some foods such as nuts, peanuts, shellfish, strawberries and coconut oils.

Signals of Anaphylaxis

Anaphylaxis usually occurs suddenly, within seconds or minutes after contact with the substance. The skin or area of the body that comes in contact with the substance usually swells and turns red (Fig. 14-1). Other signals include hives, itching, rash, weakness, nausea, stomach cramps, vomiting, dizziness and trouble breathing that includes coughing and wheezing. This trouble breathing can progress to an obstructed airway as the lips, tongue, throat and larynx (voice box) swell. Low blood pressure and shock may accompany these reactions.

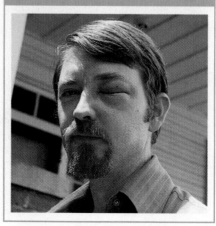

FIGURE 14-1 In anaphylaxis, the face and air passages can swell, restricting breathing.

Death from anaphylaxis may occur because the person's breathing is severely restricted.

Care for Anaphylaxis

If you notice an unusual inflammation or rash on a person's skin just after he or she has come into contact with a possible antigen, the person may be having an allergic reaction. If you suspect anaphylaxis—

- Check the person's airway and breathing.
- Call 9-1-1 or the local emergency number immediately if you find the person is having trouble breathing or if the person complains that his or her throat is closing.
- Help the person into the most comfortable position for breathing.
- Administer oxygen if it is available and you are trained to do so.
- Monitor the ABCs (airway, breathing and circulation) and try to keep the person calm.

People who know they are extremely allergic to certain substances usually try to avoid them, although this is sometimes impossible. These people may carry an anaphylaxis kit in case they have a severe reaction (Fig. 14-2). Such kits, which are available by prescription only, contain a single dose of the drug *epinephrine* that can be injected into the body to counteract the anaphylactic reaction (Fig. 14-3). Many kits also contain an *antihistamine*, a substance that reduces the effects of compounds released by the body in allergic reactions, in a pill form.

Auto-Injectors. An auto-injector contains a preloaded dose of 0.3 mg of epinephrine for adults or 0.15 mg of epinephrine for children. It is also commonly called an *Epi-Pen®*. The injector has a spring-loaded plunger that when activated injects the epi-

HEART MAY POUND AFTER INJECTION

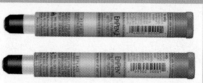

FIGURE 14-2 Anaphylaxis kits contain a single dose of the drug epinephrine, which is preloaded into an auto-injector, commonly called an Epi-Pen®.

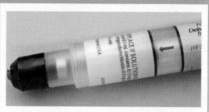

FIGURE 14-3 Used auto-injector.

nephrine. Forcefully pushing the auto-injector against the skin activates the device. It should be used on a person's upper arm or thigh in the muscular area. This injector needs to stay in place for 10 seconds to allow the medication to fully empty.

If a person is conscious and able to use the auto-injector, help him or her in any way asked. Call 9-1-1 or the local emergency number. If someone reacts so severely to a specific antigen that a physician has prescribed an epinephrine auto-injector, then the person might need advanced medical care and time is of the essence. If you know that a person has a prescribed auto-injector and is unable to administer it him- or herself, then you may help the person use it.

ASSISTANCE WITH AN EPINEPHRINE AUTO-INJECTOR

To assist with the administration of an epinephrine auto-injector, follow these steps—

Check the scene and the person. Identify yourself and ask the person if you can help.

1. Monitor the ABCs.

If the person is unconscious, has trouble breathing, complains of the throat tightening, or explains that he or she is subject to severe allergic reactions, have someone call 9-1-1 or the local emergency number.

2. Give care for life-threatening emergencies.
3. Check a conscious person to determine—
   - The substance (antigen) involved.
   - The route of exposure to the antigen.
   - The effects of the exposure.

If the person is conscious and can talk, ask—

- What is your name?
- What happened?
- How do you feel?
- Do you feel any tingling in your hands, feet or lips?
- Do you feel pain anywhere?
- Do you have any allergies? Do you have prescribed medications to take in case of an allergic reaction?
- Do you know what triggered the reaction?
- How much and how long were you exposed?
- Do you have any medical conditions or are you taking any medications?

Check the person from head to toe. **Visually inspect the body—**

- Observe for signals of respiratory distress or allergic reactions.
- Look for a medical ID tag.

Check the person's head.

- Look for swelling of the face, neck or tongue.
- Notice if the person is drowsy, not alert, confused or exhibiting slurred speech.

Check skin appearance. Look at person's face and lips.

Ask yourself, is the skin—

- Cold or hot?
- Unusually wet or dry?
- Pale, bluish or flushed?

Check the chest

- Ask if he or she is experiencing pain during breathing.
- Notice rate, depth of breaths, wheezes or gasping sounds.

Care for respiratory distress

- Help person to rest in a comfortable position, usually sitting.
- Make sure someone has called 9-1-1 or the local emergency number.
- Calm and reassure the person.

4. Document any changes in condition over time.

Assisting with an Epinephrine Auto-Injector

Determine whether the person has already taken epinephrine or antihistamine. If so, DO NOT administer another dose unless directed by EMS.

Check the label to confirm that the prescription of the auto-injector is for this person.

Check the expiration date of the auto-injector. If it has expired, DO NOT USE IT. If the medication is visible, confirm that the liquid is clear and not cloudy. If it is cloudy, DO NOT USE IT.

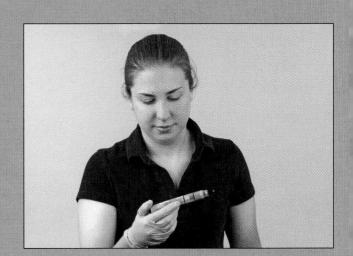

After checking a conscious person...

STEP 1

Locate the middle of one thigh or the upper arm to use as the injection site.

Grasp the auto-injector firmly in your fist, and pull off the safety cap with your other hand.

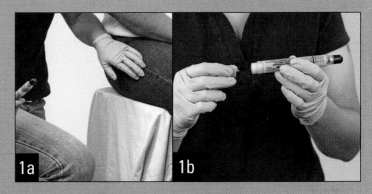

STEP 2

Hold the (black) tip (needle end) near the person's outer thigh so that the auto-injector is at a 90-degree angle to the thigh.

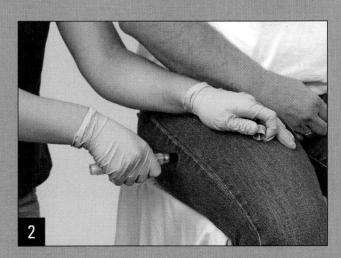

STEP 3

Swing out then firmly jab the tip straight into the outer thigh. You will hear a click.

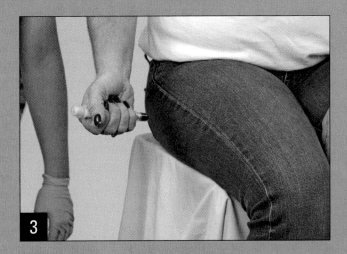

NOTE: If possible, help the person self-administer the auto-injector.

STEP 4

Hold the auto-injector firmly in place for 10 seconds, then remove it from the thigh and massage the injection site for several seconds.

Note: Recheck the person's airway, breathing and circulation and observe his or her response to the epinephrine.

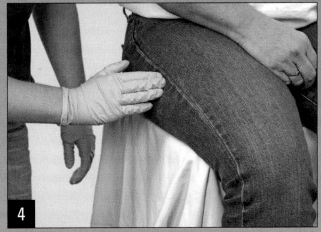

STEP 5

Give the used auto-injector to the emergency medical services personnel when they arrive.

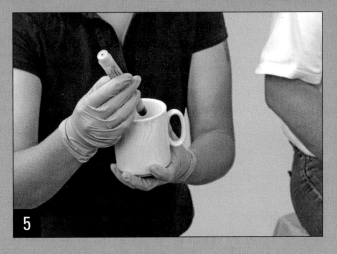

Sources

Aetna Intelihealth: *Health news*, 10 February 2002.
www.intelihealth.com/IH/ihtIH/WSIHW000/333/7228/345756.html. Accessed 12/5/2005.

American Heart Association: *Early aspirin provides quick benefits for acute stroke patients*, 2 June 2000.
www.americanheart.org. Accessed 12/5/2005.

American Heart Association: *Facts about high blood pressure, stroke, and heart profilers*, 28 April 2003.
www.americanheart.org/presenter.jhtml?identifier=3011372. Accessed 12/5/2005.

American Heart Association: *Heart disease and stroke statistics-2004 update*.
www.americanheart.org. Accessed 12/5/2005.

American Heart Association: *Stroke 2004*.
stroke.ahajournals.org/cgi/content/full/35/6/1355. Accessed 12/5/2005.

American Heart Association: *Stroke Journal Report*, 18 February 2003.
www.americanheart.org/presenter.jhtml?identifier=3008841. Accessed 12/5/2005.

American Heart Association: *Stroke: What causes a stroke?*
www.americanheart.org/presenter.jhtml?identifier=4755. Accessed 12/5/2005.

Centers for Disease Control and Prevention: *Injury fact book*.
www.cdc.gov/ncipc/fact_book/07_Different.htm. Accessed 12/5/2005.

Centers for Disease Control and Prevention, *Morbidity and Mortality Weekly Report: Surveillance Summaries 2001*.
webappa.cdc.gov/cgi-bin/broker.exe. Accessed 12/5/2005.

Centers for Disease Control and Prevention, National Agricultural Safety Database: *Venomous snake bites*, Palm
Beach Herpetological Society and the University of Florida: Institute of Food and Agricultural Sciences, April 2004.
www.cdc.gov/nasd/docs/d000001-d000100/d000054/d000054.html. Accessed 12/5/2005.

Centers for Disease Control and Prevention, National Center for Health Care Statistics: *Life expectancy health stats*.
www.cdc.gov/nchs/fastats/lifexpec.htm. Accessed 12/5/2005.

Centers for Disease Control and Prevention, National Center for Health Care Statistics: *News release 1998*.
www.cdc.gov/nchs/pressroom/98news/huspr98.htm. Accessed 12/5/2005.

Centers for Disease Control and Prevention: *National vital statistics report*. 7 March 2005.
www.cdc.gov/nchs/fastats/pdf/Pages%20from%20nvsr53_17t2.pdf. Accessed 12/5/2005.

Centers for Disease Control and Prevention: *Poisonings: fact sheet*.
www.cdc.gov/ncipc/factsheets/poisoning.htm. Accessed 12/5/2005.

Centers for Disease Control and Prevention: *Preventing heart disease and stroke*.
www.cdc.gov/nccdphp/bb_heartdisease/index.htm. Accessed 12/5/2005.

Centers for Disease Control and Prevention: *Spinal cord injury (SCI) fact sheet*.
www.cdc.gov/ncipc/factsheets/scifacts.htm. Accessed 12/5/2005.

Epilepsy Foundation: *Epilepsy and seizure statistics*.
www.epilepsyfoundation.org/answerplace/statistics.cfm. Accessed 12/5/2005.

Federal Citizen Information Center: *Consumer focus: water safety*.
www.pueblo.gsa.gov/cfocus/cfwatersafety04/focus2.htm. Accessed 12/5/2005.

Home Safety Council: *Home safety tips: poison safety tips*.
www.homesafetycouncil.org/safety_guide/sg_poison_w001aspx. Accessed 12/5/2005.

Home Safety Council: *Home safety tips: poison safety tips.*
www.homesafetycouncil.org/safety_guide/sg_poison_w002.aspx. Accessed 12/5/2005.

National Heart, Lung, and Blood Institute: *Diseases and conditions index.*
www.nhlbi.nih.gov /health/dci/Diseases/HeartAttack/HeartAttack_WhatIs.html. Accessed 12/5/2005.

National Highway Traffic Administration,
www.nhtsa.dot.gov/portal/site/nhtsa/menuitem.9f8c7d6359e0e9bbbf30811060008a0c/. Accessed 12/5/2005.

University of Iowa Hospitals and Clinics: *UI Health Care News*: January 3, 2005.
www.uihealthcare.com/news/news/2005/01/03accidents.html. Accessed 12/5/2005.

University of Missouri, Extension: *Missouri families' health.*
missourifamilies.org/quick/healthqa/healthqa52.htm. Accessed 12/5/2005.

Yahoo Health Osteoporosis Health Center: *You are never too young or too old to deal with Osteoporosis.*
health.yahoo.com/centers/strongbones/103. Accessed 12/5/2005.

Index

A

ABCs (airway/breathing/circulation), 19, 32-34
Abdominal injuries, 125
Abdominal thrusts, 49-51
Abnormal heart rhythm, 68
Abrasions, 113
Absorbed poisons, 163
Action plan for emergencies, 26-27
Adhesive compresses, 115, 116
Adults, defined, 30
Advance directives, 84-85
Advanced medical care in Cardiac Chain of Survival, 72
AED, 19, 68
  for adults, 80-81
  in cardiac emergencies, 71, 72
  for children, 81-82
  learning, 10
  maintenance of AEDs, 84
  precautions in using AEDs, 82-83
  skill sheets, 98-101
  special situations, 83
  types of AEDs, 81
  see also Defibrillation
Agonal breath, 33
AIDS (acquired immune deficiency syndrome), 5
  see also HIV (human immunodeficiency virus)
Air in the stomach in breathing emergencies, 55
Airway in ABCs, 32
Alcohol use and abuse, 104, 105
Allergic reactions, 199-200
  and breathing emergencies, 48
American Diabetes Association, 154, 155
Anaphylactic shock, 48
  allergic reactions, 199-200
  assistance with an auto-injector, 201-204
  auto-injectors, 200-204
  care for, 200-204
  defined, 199
  epinephrine and antihistamine, 200
  prevalence of, 199
  signals of, 48, 200
Anaphylaxis. *See* Anaphylactic shock
Anatomic splints, 135
Angina pectoris, 70
Animal bites, 5, 170-171, 172
Anti-inflammatory medications for asthma, 195
Antibiotics, 5

Antibodies, 199
Antigens, 199
Antihistamine, 200
Antitoxins, 115
Arteries, 68, 118
  blocked, 159
Aspirin
  in cardiac emergencies, 70, 71
  and children, 186
Asthma, 48, 76, 193-197
  asthma inhalers, 196-197
  defined, 193
  medications for, 195
  prevalence of, 193
  signals of an attack, 195
  triggers of, 193, 194-195
Asystole, 68
Atria, 68
Aura in epilepsy, 158
Auto-injectors for anaphylactic shock, 200-203
Automated external defibrillation. *See* AED
Avulsions, 114

B

Back blows and abdominal thrusts, 49-51
Bacteria, 5
  see also Disease
Bandage compresses, 115
Bandages, 114-115, 115-118
Barriers to action in emergencies, 3-6
Bike safety, 107
Black widow spiders, 165
Blanket drag, 25
Bleeding
  internal, 112
  severe, 34, 45, 111, 118, 126
  skill sheet for controlling bleeding, 126
Blood
  cleaning up a spill, 9
  in disease spreading, 5, 6, 54
  and HIV/AIDS, 8
Blood thinners, 70
Blood vessels, 118
Body fluids
  in disease spreading, 5, 6, 54
  and HIV/AIDS, 8
Bones, 131, 132
  see also Muscle, bone and joint injuries
Brain damage, 46, 47
Breathing barriers, protective, 6, 54-55
Breathing emergencies, 45-65
  brain damage, 46, 47

breathing barriers, 54-55
  caring for, 48-49
  child-proofing home, 56-57
  child safety IQ, 58
  conditions causing, 48
  and head, neck, and back injuries, 46, 58-59
  mouth-to-nose breathing, 55
  rescue breathing for children, 52-53
  rescue breathing for infants, 53-54
  respiratory distress and respiratory arrest, 46-47
  signals of, 47
  skill sheets, 63-65
  special situations, 55, 58-59
  for stomas, 55, 58-59
  submersion victims, 55
  trouble breathing, 47
  see also Choking emergencies; CPR
Breathing in ABCs, 32-34
Bronchitis, 48
Bronchodilators for asthma, 195
Brown recluse spiders, 165
Burns, 111, 119-121
Bystanders calling 9-1-1, 3, 4

C

Calcium, 140-141
CALL, 17-19
  Call First or Care First?, 17-19, 45, 46, 55
  see also Nine-one-one (9-1-1)
Capillaries, 118
Cardiac arrest, 19, 68, 71-72
Cardiac Chain of Survival, 72, 74
Cardiac emergencies, 67-101
  and aspirin, 70, 71
  Cardiac Chain of Survival, 72, 74
  care for heart attacks, 71-76
  in children and infants, 76-80
  heart stops beating, 71-72
  prompt action is key, 71
  signals of heart attacks, 69-71
  see also AED; CPR
Cardiopulmonary resuscitation. *See* CPR
Cardiovascular disease as cause of death, 1, 2, 67-68
CARE, 19-20
  general guidelines, 19-20
  transporting the victim, 20
Care First or Call First?, 17-19, 45, 46, 55
CDC. *See* Centers for Disease Control and Prevention
Centers for Disease Control and Prevention (CDC), 8, 48, 188, 193

CHECK
life-threatening conditions, 18
the scene for safety, 16-17
the victim, 17
CHECK/CALL/CARE (emergency action steps), 15-27, 74
Checking an ill or injured person, 29-43
ABCs, 32-34
conducting interviews, 30
conscious person, 29-32
head to toe checking, 30-32
pulse of children and infants, 33
severe bleeding, 34
shock, 34-35
skill sheets, 36-43
unconscious infant, 29
unconscious person, 29, 32-34
see also Emergency action steps (CHECK/CALL/CARE)
Chemical burns, 120
Chemical poisoning, 165
Chest compressions in CPR, 74-75
Chest injuries, 123, 138-139
Chest thrusts in choking emergencies, 50
Child abuse, 186
Childbirth, 188
Children
breathing emergencies in, 47
car safety seats, 105
cardiac emergencies in, 76-80
checking and caring for in emergencies, 17
child abuse, 186
child-proofing home, 56-57
child safety IQ, 58
choking in conscious, 49-50
CPR for, 76-78
defined, 30
injuries in, 2
injury and illness, 185-186
poisoning, 161, 186
preventing choking, 52
pulses of, 33
rescue breathing for, 52-53
unconscious, 19
unconscious choking, 79, 88-89, 92-93
see also Infants
Choking emergencies, 49-52, 53
back blows and abdominal thrusts, 49-51
care for, 49
causes of, 53
chest thrusts in, 50
child-proofing home, 56-57
child safety IQ, 58
conscious adult or child, 49-50
conscious infants, 51-52
preventing choking in children and

infants, 52
skill sheets, 60-62
special situations, 50
unconscious choking adult or child, 79, 88-89, 92-93
unconscious choking infant, 79-80, 96-97
universal signal, 49
see also Breathing emergencies
Cholesterol, 73, 157
Chronic conditions, 153
Cigarette smoking, 73, 157
Circulation in ABCs, 34
Closed fractures, 132
Closed wounds, 112-113
Clothes drag, 25
Clothing for cold weather, 181
Cold-related illness, 178-180
see also Heat- and cold-related emergencies
Common cold, 5
Conscious person
checking a, 29-32
choking in, 49-50
Consent to give care, 9
Convulsions, 156
Copperhead snakes, 169
Coral snakes, 169-170
Coronary heart disease, 67-68
deaths from, 73
heart healthy IQ, 80
preventing, 73
see also Cardiovascular disease
Cottonmouth snakes, 169
Coumadin, 70
CPR, 18
for adults, 74-75, 77
in cardiac emergencies, 68, 71, 72
chest compressions, 74-75
for children, 76-78
for infants, 76, 77, 78-79
learning, 10
moving victim to perform, 20
skill sheets, 86-87, 90-91, 94-95
two responders available, 75
when to give, 33, 46
when to stop, 76
see also Breathing emergencies
Crime scenes and hostile situations, 191

D

Deaths
from cardiovascular disease, 1, 2, 67-68
from diabetes, 154
from injuries, 103, 104
leading causes of, 1
from poisoning, 161
Deciding to act in emergencies, 3-6

Deer ticks, 166-167
DEET, 168
Defibrillation, 68, 72
see also AED
Degenerative diseases, 153
Diabetes, 153-156
and stroke, 158
Diet and stroke, 157-158
Disability
defined, 188
see also People with disabilities
Disease
degenerative, 153
prevention of transmission, 4, 6, 54
spread of, 4, 5
see also Cardiovascular disease
Disks, 137
Dislocations, 132-133
Dispatchers, 19
Disposable gloves, 6
removing, 12-13
Diuretics, 175
DNR. See "Do Not Resuscitate"
"Do Not Resuscitate" (DNR), 85
Dressings, 114-115
Drowning, 19, 55, 105
Drug overdoses, 19, 161, 162
Durable powers of attorney for health care, 84-85

E
Elastic roller bandages, 117-118
Elderly. See Older adults
Electrical burns, 121
Electrical impulses, 130
Embedded objects, 121-122
Emergencies, 1-13
barriers to action, 3-6
calling 9-1-1, 6
deciding to act, 3-6
developing an action plan, 26-27
getting consent to give care, 9
giving care until help arrives, 9
Good Samaritan laws, 6
life-threatening conditions, 18, 45
reaching and moving an ill or injured person, 20-25
recognizing, 2-3
see also Breathing emergencies; Moving an ill or injured person
Emergency action steps (CHECK/CALL/CARE), 15-27
CALL, 17-19
CARE, 19-20
CHECK, 16-17
Emergency kits. See First aid kits
Emergency medical care, 19

Emergency medical services (EMS) system, 2, 4
Emergency number. *See* Nine-one-one (9-1-1)
Emphysema, 48
EMS. *See* Emergency medical services (EMS) system
Epilepsy, 156
Epinephrine and antihistamine, 200
Eye and foot safety, 107

F
Face shields, 54-55
    see also Breathing barriers
Fainting, 152-153
FAST (face/arm/speech/time) in stroke, 158
FCC. *See* Federal Communications Commission
FDA. *See* Food and Drug Administration
Febrile seizures, 156
Federal Communications Commission (FCC), 21
Federal Patient Self-Determination Act, 84
Fire safety, 105-106
First aid kits, 6, 10, 11
    contents of, 22
First-degree burns (superficial), 120, 121
    see also Soft tissue injuries
Food and Drug Administration (FDA), 159
Foot drag, 25
Fractures, 131-132, 133
Frostbite, 178, 179

G
Gloves. *See* Disposable gloves
Good Samaritan laws, 6
Ground splints, 136

H
H.A.IN.E.S. (High Arm Endangered Spine) position, 46
Hand washing, 6
Head, neck, and back injuries, 136-138
    and breathing emergencies, 46, 58-59
    H.A.IN.E.S. (High Arm Endangered Spine) position, 46
Head-tilt/chin-lift technique, 32, 33
Head to toe checking, 30-32
Health-care surrogate or proxy, 85
Hearing loss, 189-190
Heart
    description and diagram, 67
    failure of, 68-69
    see also Cardiac emergencies; Cardiovascular disease
Heart attacks. *See* Cardiac emergencies
Heart disease. *See* Cardiovascular disease; Coronary heart disease

Heat- and cold-related emergencies, 175-181
    clothing for cold weather, 181
    cold-related illness, 178-180
    heat-related illness, 177-178
    illnesses from, 175, 176
    older adults, 188
    people at risk for, 175
    preventing, 180, 181
    signals of, 175
Heat cramps, 177
Heat exhaustion, 177
Heat-related illness, 177-178
    see also Heat- and cold-related emergencies
Heat stroke, 177-178
Hepatitis B virus (HBV), 5
Hepatitis C virus (HBC), 5
Herpes simplex II virus, 5
High blood pressure, 73, 157
HIV (human immunodeficiency virus), 5
    hotline, 8
    testing, 8
    transmission during first aid, 8
    see also AIDS (acquired immune deficiency syndrome)
Home escape plan, 106
Home safety, 106-107
Hostile situations, 191
Hotel escape plan, 105
Hyperglycemia, 154
Hyperventilation, 48
Hypoglycemia, 154
Hypothermia, 178-180
Hypothermia and AED, 83

I
ICD. *See* Implantable cardioverter-defibrillator
Illness. *See* Sudden illness
Immune system, 199
Implantable cardioverter-defibrillator (ICD), 83
Implantable devices and AED, 83
Infants
    breathing emergencies in, 47
    car safety seats, 105
    cardiac emergencies in, 76-80
    checking unconscious, 29
    child abuse, 186
    child-proofing home, 56-57
    child safety IQ, 58
    choking in conscious, 51-52
    CPR for, 76, 77, 78-79
    defined, 30
    injury and illness, 185-186
    preventing choking, 52
    pulses of, 33

    rescue breathing for, 53-54
    sudden infant death syndrome (SIDS), 186
    unconscious choking in, 79-80, 96-97
    see also Children
Infection, 111, 113
Inhaled poisons, 162, 163
Injected poisons, 163
Injuries
    as cause of death, 1, 2, 103, 104
    see also Injury prevention; Muscle, bone and joint injuries; Soft tissue injuries
Injury prevention, 103-109
    alcohol use and abuse, 104, 105
    bike safety, 107
    deaths from injuries, 103, 104
    eye and foot safety, 107
    fire safety, 105-106
    home escape plan, 106
    home safety, 106-107
    hotel escape plan, 105
    play safety, 107-108
    protective devices, 104
    reducing risk for injury, 104-105
    risk factors for injury, 104
    running safety, 108
    survey, 109
    swimming safety, 107-108
    vehicle safety, 105
    water safety, 107-108
    work safety, 107
    see also Muscle, bone and joint injuries; Soft tissue injuries
Insect bites and stings, 165, 172
Insect repellents, 168, 169
Insulin, 154
    see also Diabetes
Insurance records, 10
Internal bleeding, 112
Interviewing the victim, 30
Ischemic stroke, 159

J
Jellyfish, 171
Joints, 131, 132
    see also Muscle, bone and joint injuries
Junk food, 73

L
Lacerations, 114
Language barriers, 190-191
Lawsuits, 7
Lay responders, 7
Life-threatening conditions, 18, 45
Ligaments, 130, 131
Lip injuries, 122
Lip reading, 189

Living wills, 84-85
Local emergency numbers, 10
   see also Nine-one-one (9-1-1)
Lyme disease, 166-167

M

Marine life, poisonings from, 171, 172
Medicaid, 84
Medical ID tags, 10, 32, 48, 153
Medical information, 10, 11
Medicare, 84
Mental impairment, 190
Merci device, 159
Mosquitoes, 168
Motor function, 189
Motor impairment, 190
Mouth injuries, 122
Mouth-to-nose breathing, 55
Moving an ill or injured person, 20-25
   blanket drag, 25
   clothes drag, 25
   foot drag, 25
   pack-strap carry, 23-24
   two-person seat carry, 24
   walking assist, 22-23
Muscle, bone, and joint injuries, 129-149
   bones, 131, 132
   caring for, 135-136
      RICE (rest/immobilize/cold/elevate),
       135
      splinting, 135-136
   chest injuries, 138-139
   head, neck, and back injuries, 136-138
   joints, 131, 132
   muscles, 130-131
   osteoporosis, 140-141
   pelvic injuries, 139
   signals of serious injuries, 133,
      134-135
   skill sheets for splints, 142-149
   types of injuries, 131-139
      dislocations, 132-133
      fractures, 131-132, 133
      sprains, 133, 134
      strains, 133-134

N

Nine-one-one (9-1-1)
   bystanders calling, 3, 4, 45
   local emergency numbers, 10
   talking to dispatcher, 19
   when to call, 6, 7, 9, 17-19, 20, 45,
      46, 152
   wireless, 21
   see also CALL
Nitroglycerin patches and AED, 83
Nose injuries, 122

O

Occlusive dressings, 115
Older adults, 186-188
   checking and caring for in emergencies,
      17, 187
   confusion in, 187-188
   falls, 187
   head injuries, 187
   heat and cold problems, 188
Open fractures, 132
Open wounds, 113-119
Osteoporosis, 131, 140-141
Overweight, 73
Oxygen, 68

P

Pack-strap carry, 23-24
Paralysis, 130, 137
Parents and caregivers, 184-185
Pelvic injuries, 139
People with disabilities, 188-190
   hearing loss, 189-190
   mental impairment, 190
   motor impairment, 190
   physical disabilities, 189
   vision loss, 190
Physical disabilities, 189
Physical exercise, 73, 140-141
Plan of action for emergencies, 26-27
Plant poisonings, 171-173
Play safety, 107-108
Poison Control Centers, 10, 106, 161,
   164
Poison ivy, 173
Poison oak, 173
Poison sumac, 173
Poisoning, 161-173
   absorbed poisons, 163
   in adults, 161
   animals, 170-171, 172
   caring for bites and stings, 172
   checking the scene, 163-164
   in children, 161
   deaths from, 161
   defined, 161
   general care guidelines, 164
   inhaled poisons, 162, 163
   injected poisons, 163
   insects, 165, 172
   Lyme disease, 166-167
   marine life, 171, 172
   mosquitoes, 168
   plants, 171-173
   Poison Control Centers, 10, 106, 161, 164
   prevalence of, 161
   preventing, 163, 173
   preventing bites and stings, 170

   scorpions and spiders, 165, 169, 172
   signals of, 164
   snakes, 169-170, 172
   substance abuse, 162
   swallowed poisons, 162, 163
   toxic fumes, 164
   West Nile Virus (WNV), 168
   wet and dry chemicals, 165
Portuguese man-of-war, 171
Pregnant women, chest thrusts in choking
   emergencies, 50
Pressure bandages, 115
Protective breathing barriers, 6
Protective devices, 104
Public Service Answering Point, 21
Pulses of children and infants, 33
Puncture wounds, 114
   in the chest, 123-124

R

Rabies, 170-171
Radiation (sun) burns, 121
Rattlesnakes, 169
Recovery positions, 46
Recreation safety, 107-108
Rescue breathing, 33, 46
   for children, 52-53
   for infants, 53-54
   see also Breathing emergencies
Respiratory distress and respiratory arrest,
   46-47
   see also Breathing emergencies; CPR
Resuscitation masks, 54-55
   see also Breathing barriers
Reye's syndrome, 186
Rib fractures, 123
RICE (rest/immobilize/cold/elevate), 135
Rigid splints, 136
Roller bandages, 115-118
Running safety, 108

S

Safety. *See* Injury prevention
Saturated fats, 73, 157
Scene
   checking for safety, 16-17, 18
   immediate danger, 20
Scorpions, 165, 169
Sea anemone, 171
Second-degree burns (partial thickness),
   119, 120
   see also Soft tissue injuries
Seizures, 156-157
Severed body parts, 121
Shock
   caring for, 34-35
   signals of, 34

SIDS. *See* Sudden infant death syndrome
Sign language, 189
Skill sheets
  AED in adults, 98-99
  AED in children, 100-101
  assisting with an asthma inhaler, 196-197
  assisting with an epinephrine auto-
      injector, 202-204
  controlling external bleeding, 126
  checking a conscious person, 36-38
  checking an unconscious adult, 39
  checking an unconscious child, 40-41
  checking an unconscious infant, 42-43
  conscious choking in adults, 60
  conscious choking in children, 61
  conscious choking in infants, 62
  CPR for adults, 86-87
  CPR in children, 90-91
  CPR in infants, 94-95
  removing gloves, 12-13
  how to give a rescue breath in adults, 63
  rescue breathing in children, 64
  rescue breathing in infants, 65
  applying a sling and binder, 148-149
  applying an anatomic splint, 142-143
  applying a rigid splint, 146-147
  applying a soft splint, 144-145
  unconscious choking in adults, 88-89
  unconscious choking in children, 92-93
  unconscious choking in infants, 96-97
Smoke alarms, 105
Smoking, 73, 157
Snakes, 169-170, 172
Soft splints, 135-136
Soft tissue injuries, 111-126
  abdominal injuries, 125
  bandages, 114-115
  burns, 111, 119-121
    caring for, 120-121
    critical burns, 119
    preventing, 121
    sources of, 119, 120-121
    types of, 119, 120
  chest injuries, 123
    puncture wounds, 123-124
    rib fractures, 123
    sucking chest wounds, 124-125
  dressings, 114-115
  embedded objects, 121-122
  infection, 111, 113
  internal bleeding, 112
  lip injuries, 122
  mouth injuries, 122
  nose injuries, 122
  severe bleeding, 111, 118, 126
  severed body parts, 121

  skill sheet for controlling bleeding, 126
  soft tissues defined, 111
  stitches, 116
  tetanus, 115
  tooth injuries, 122-123
  wounds, 112-119
    closed wounds, 112-113
    open wounds, 113-119
  see also Injury prevention
Special situations and circumstances,
      183-191
  childbirth, 188
  crime scenes and hostile situations, 191
  infants and children, 183-186
  language barriers, 190-191
  older adults, 186-188
  people with disabilities, 188-190
Spiders, 165, 169
Spine, 137
Splinting, 135-136, 142-149
Sprains, 133, 134
Stingray, 171
Stitches, 116
Stomas, rescue breathing for, 55, 58-59
Strains, 133-134
Streptococcus agalactia bacteria, 5
Stroke, 157-159
  care for, 159
  FAST (face/arm/speech/time), 158
  prevention of, 158
  risk factors, 157-158
  signals of, 158-159
  thrombolytic drugs ("clot-busters"),
      159
Strokes as cause of death, 2, 68
Submersion victims
  breathing emergencies in, 55
  see also Drowning
Substance abuse, 162
Sucking chest wounds, 124-125
Sudden illness, 151-159
  caring for, 152, 159
  chronic conditions, 153
  diabetes, 153-156
  fainting, 152-153
  seizures, 156-157
  signals of, 151-152
  stroke, 157-159
  when to call 9-1-1, 152
Sudden infant death syndrome (SIDS),
      186
Suicide, 161
Sunburn, 121
Swallowed poisons, 162, 163
Swimming safety, 107-108

T
TDD. *See* Telecommunications device for
      the deaf
Telecommunications device for the deaf
      (TDD), 189
Tendons, 130
Tetanus, 115
Third-degree burns (full thickness), 119,
      120
  see also Soft tissue injuries
Thrombolytic drugs ("clot-busters"), 159
Ticks, 166-167
Tooth injuries, 122-123
Toxic fumes, 164
Trauma and AED, 83
Two-person seat carry, 24

U
Unconscious persons, 45
  checking, 29, 32-34
  checking infants, 29
  choking adult or child, 79, 88-89, 92-93
  choking infants, 79-80, 96-97
Unintentional injury, 104
  see also Injury prevention; Muscle, bone
      and joint injuries; Soft tissue
      injuries
Universal signal for choking, 49

V
Vehicle safety, 105
Veins, 118
Ventricles, 68
Ventricular fibrillation (V-fib), 68
Ventricular tachycardia (V-tach), 68
Vertebrae, 137
Viruses, 5
  see also Disease
Vision loss, 190
Vitamin D, 140-141
Vomiting
  in breathing emergencies, 46, 55
  in sudden illnesses, 159

W
Walking assist, 22-23
Warfarin, 70
Washing hands, 6
Water safety, 107-108
West Nile Virus (WNV), 168
Wet environments and AED, 83
Wills, living, 84-85
Wireless (9-1-1), 21
Work safety, 107
Wounds, 112-119